What Are You Afraid Of?

What Are You Afraid Of?

A Body/Mind Guide to Courageous Living

LAVINIA PLONKA

Jeremy P. Tarcher/Penguin

a member of Penguin Group (USA) Inc. New York

JEREMY P. TARCHER/PENGUIN
Published by the Penguin Group
www.penguin.com
Penguin Group (USA) Inc., 375 Hudson Street, New York, New York 10014, USA • Penguin
Group (Canada), 10 Alcorn Avenue, Toronto, Ontario M4V 3B2, Canada (a division of Pearson
Penguin Canada Inc.) • Penguin Books Ltd, 80 Strand, London WC2R 0RL, England
• Penguin Ireland, 25 St Stephen's Green, Dublin 2, Ireland (a division of Penguin Books Ltd)
• Penguin Group (Australia), 250 Camberwell Road, Camberwell, Victoria 3124, Australia
(a division of Pearson Australia Group Pty Ltd) • Penguin Books India Pvt Ltd, 11 Community
Centre, Panchsheel Park, New Delhi–110 017, India • Penguin Group (NZ), cnr Airborne and
Rosedale Roads, Albany, Auckland 1310, New Zealand (a division of Pearson New Zealand Ltd.)
• Penguin Books (South Africa) (Pty) Ltd, 24 Sturdee Avenue, Rosebank, Johannesburg
2196, South Africa

Penguin Books Ltd, Registered Offices: 80 Strand, London, WC2R 0RL, England

First trade paperback edition 2005
Copyright © 2004 by Lavinia Plonka
Illustrations by Ron Morecraft

While the author has made every effort to provide accurate telephone numbers and Internet addresses at the time of publication, neither the publisher nor the author assumes any responsibility
for errors, or for changes that occur after publication.

Every effort has been made to ensure that the information contained in this book is complete
and accurate. However, neither the publisher nor the author is engaged in rendering professional
advice or services to the individual reader. The ideas, procedures, and suggestions contained in this
book are not intended as a subsitute for consulting with your physician. All matters regarding
your health require medical supervision. Neither the author nor the publisher shall be liable or
responsible for any loss or damage allegedly arising from any information or suggestion in this
book.

Unless otherwise indicated, the names and circumstances of the people in the case studies and
anecdotes have all been changed.

Most Tarcher/Penguin books are available at special quantity discounts for bulk purchase for sales
promotions, premiums, fund-raising, and educational needs. Special books or book excerpts also can
be created to fit specific needs. For details, write Penguin Group (USA) Inc. Special Markets, 375
Hudson Street, New York, NY 10014.

The Library of Congress cataloged the hardcover edition as follows:

Plonka, Lavinia.
What are you afraid of?: a body/mind guide to courageous living / Lavinia Plonka.
    p.   cm.
Includes bibliographical references and index.
ISBN 1-58542-285-1
1. Feldenkrais method.   2. Fear.   I. Title.
RC489.F44P565   2004   2003064567
616.7'0622—dc22

ISBN 1-58542-393-9 (paperback edition)

Printed in the United States of America

1   3   5   7   9   10   8   6   4   2

Book design by Kate Nichols

Acknowledgments

This book would not have happened without the inspiration of Reverend Mary Marcus, the editing of Mitch Horowitz, and the support of the women in my writers' group.

To Ron—

The mirror of my fondest hopes

and my deepest fears

Contents

Part III. *Tools and Activities*

What Are You Afraid Of?

Introduction: Me? Afraid?

The person walking toward me on a crowded Manhattan street. Making the phone call for that new business idea. Telling my mother to stop meddling in my brother's affairs. Quitting my job. Telling my husband what I need in bed. Joining the environmental group that's fighting the land developer who happens to be my wife's colleague. Going to the doctor. Deciding to change doctors. Letting my child travel alone. The person walking *behind* me on a deserted Manhattan street. Missing the plane. Being wrong. The list could go on for pages. We are constantly afraid.

Drive down any highway in America and sooner or later you'll see it. It's a decal stuck on the back window that says NO FEAR! What does it mean, really, to be free of fear? The philosopher and spiritual teacher Krishnamurti once said that there are only two emotions: love and fear. Every other emotion grows out of this pair of basic, primal feelings. Now, of course, we all want to feel bathed in love, but it seems more often we find ourselves sitting with fear's relatives: insecurity, pride, anger, territorialism, to name a few.

Of course, fear is a useful emotion. In *Body and Mature Behavior*, Dr. Moshe Feldenkrais, a pioneering researcher in the field of movement studies, observed that infants are "practically insensitive to external stimuli"—except for the fear of falling. In the face of perceived danger, an infant contracts its muscles and holds its breath, which becomes the adult fear response. This innate protective mechanism was designed by nature to help us survive.

It's wise to feel a little apprehension while approaching a tiger, or driving a hairpin turn along the Amalfi coast. It sharpens the mechanism's response time, enhances alertness, speeds escape if necessary. But somewhere in man's development, fear has turned into a constant companion.

Life has never been more secure, really, for many people in the world. Our power over nature has never been greater, in every way—and yet we've never been so uneasy. The Bushmen in the Kalahari—who had none of the things we have, where life was the ancient life of the hunter, unpredictable and dangerous—felt more secure than we feel in the midst of our plenty, alone at night in our beds.   —SIR LAURENS VAN DER POST

It Really *Is* Chemical

When fear grips you, the brain fires neurotransmitters that shoot adrenaline and other chemicals through your entire body. We all know the physical sensation—sweaty palms, changed breathing pattern, increased heart rate—also known as the "fight-or-flight" response. These sensations signal the system to run for cover, to protect itself. The digestive process shuts down; blood runs to the legs. All of these reactions put stress on the entire organism. Over a lifetime, they can affect health, self-esteem, and, eventually, well-being. Carolyn Myss wrote in *Anatomy of the Spirit,* "As our lives unfold, our biological health becomes a living, breathing biographical statement that conveys our strengths, weaknesses, hopes and fears." In other words, your biography *is* your biology.

The fight-or-flight signal is firing constantly—from the moment you merge onto the highway at 65 mph into rush hour traffic while trying to negotiate your grande latte, to the sound of your boss's footsteps coming toward your cubicle, to the phone ringing twenty minutes *after* you expected your daughter home. The level of anxiety in our culture has sent our nervous systems into a tailspin, leaving many professionals feeling that pharmaceuticals are the only solution, flooding the market with antianxiety drugs that are supposed to make our lives "normal." According to a report by the University of Ottawa, 87 million people world-wide suffer from anxiety disorders. The report also stated that sales of antianxiety drugs in 1999 totaled $2 billion, with projected sales of $3 billion for 2009.

In working with hundreds of people through the years, I have seen that behind much disease, pain, and psychological paralysis, the culprit is fear. Often the fear is something residual from childhood that has become frozen in a posture—perhaps hunched shoulders, or a constant "deer in the headlights" expression. Something as simple as fear of falling can become such a phobia that a person is literally immobilized in certain situations. And it's just one letter to change fear of *falling* to fear of *failing*. Fear is often the process of taking a past negative experience and posing it as a potential future negative experience.

While governed by fear, there is no present—only negative memories and anxiety about the future. You can take drugs, but, until you learn to listen to the deep voices of fear in your cells, you will merely be masking the inner trembling that plagues your progress and stilts your development.

Fear can take many forms—from defensive reactions to criticism to out-and-out phobias. Sometimes even daredevil behavior, like skydiving, is an unconscious counterphobic choice. Many times, you don't even know that you are afraid, let alone what you are afraid of. Fear is so much a part of human wiring that it's impossible to see, like a blind spot. That's why you can talk and analyze till you're blue in the face, but if fear courses through your veins it doesn't hear the rational mind telling it to go away.

I once had a conversation with an acquaintance. Her husband had recently told her that he was having an affair, and that he was dissatisfied with their relationship. It was obvious that she was in severe pain, and desperately afraid of her imminent abandonment. She kept saying to me, "I just have to fill my life with light and love. If I keep putting love in my heart, everything will be just fine. Everything will be just fine."

Of course, it was not fine, and it didn't end up fine either. Her words were just that . . . words. That's not to say that words don't help. They have a power to heal or destroy as well. But the body and the intellect have to work together to create the life you want. After all, as was said earlier, your experiences are recorded not just in your mental memories but in your cells, in your movements, and in your posture. Working directly with the body can bypass analysis, blame, and false memories. Your movements can provide the keys to unlocking your own personal dance of fear as well as practical tools for finding courageous alternatives. By learning to recognize the "habit" of fear in your everyday movements, you can begin to remove the obstacles between yourself and the life you want. Studying your physical postures, reactions, and tensions is a direct approach to this goal.

What Are You Afraid Of? is the result of my personal journey to understand fear in myself, as well as in my practice with others. My work centers around what is called "somatic education"—learning through movement and studying the body/mind relationship to the world. Thirty years ago, I began a career as a movement artist, studying classical theater techniques like mime, mask, and clown. Concurrently, I became a student of yoga and dove deeply into several spiritual traditions. As my teaching career developed, I noticed the healing properties of theater and began using them outside the performance arena—from personal development workshops to helping inner-city children with self-esteem issues. Around that time, I became aware of the field of somatic education. After some experimentation, I embarked on a four-year training to become a Feldenkrais® practitioner.

For over ten years now, I have taught classes to the general public and worked with hundreds of individuals to help improve the quality of their lives. Many of my students came to me with severe pain, both physical and emotional. Many had been through the traditional medicine route and/or had spent a great deal of time and money in therapy, to no avail. In our work together, we often discovered that working with movement went directly, yet safely, to the habits surrounding a physical or psychological issue. Many times, the difficulties were connected to fear. The Courageous Living workshops evolved out of these discoveries.

My wish is to provide you with the tools to step forward and present your true self to the world using love, not fear, as the road to realization. Each one of us possesses everything we need to be who we were meant to be. Locked inside each paralyzed heart is enough love to save the world. The key is in your possession: It's your very own body.

Part I
The Roots of Fear

1. *Addicted to Fear*

Fear lurks in the snapping retort made to a well-meaning colleague, in the unconscious hunching of your shoulders as you slam on your brakes, in the shallow breaths you take as you listen to your child's teacher talk about his acting out. What was designed by nature to help you survive has become a liability. In this chapter, we'll explore why.

Learning to Fear

We are creatures of habit. After all, if you didn't have habits, then every day you'd have to relearn how to brush your teeth, think before you grind the coffee (and who can do that?), ponder before hitting the brakes to avoid an accident. Needless to say, you might never get out of the house, and you'd certainly never make it to work. The human organism is a complex learning system, constantly taking information in, processing it, and adding it to the functioning being. The way you respond to other stimuli is habitual as well. If every time you brought home an art project from school your mother threw it away without looking at it, you'd develop the habit of believing that your work has no value. This becomes part of your system. When you touch the flame of a match a couple of times, and learn that this is hot, you develop a habit of avoiding flames. Sometimes habits evolve that are not so linear. One child whose father constantly waved her through the air playing airplane may develop a fear of heights, another may become a skydiver. There are many factors surrounding every impression we receive.

Studies have shown that an infant begins learning in the womb, developing muscle responses to the mother's phonemes. While an animal is born with the *instinct* to walk or climb within hours, sometimes even minutes after birth, by contrast the human child learns almost everything. Those grimaces the newborn makes are the first attempts at trying to imitate the parents' expressions. A human's approach to survival is to adapt. Thus, a child whose father limps can develop a ghost limp. The reasoning is primitive: If I walk like Daddy, he won't throw me out in the cold. Antonio Damasio, in his book *Descartes' Error,* states that even qualities like altruism are learned survival strategies and not the manifestation of higher evolution. "Altruistic behavior . . . saves altruists from the future pain and suffering that would have been caused by loss or shame upon not behaving altruistically."

So a child may learn that being nice and helping people help him gain social status, assuring him survival. This behavior develops into a habit that becomes "hardwired" in the system; and the child grows up to run an inner-city health clinic, or, more likely, becomes overly obsequious trying to please everyone. It's that person's habitual approach to survival.

So what does altruism have to do with fear? Well, fear gets hardwired right in there with our survival strategy. And then it becomes, as Feldenkrais labeled it, parasitic. Let's say Daddy always used to say your finest quality was how nice you are to everyone. Not your poems, not your ballet dancing. Your child mind decides you are no good at poetry, so you refine the art of being nice to such a high degree that when you wake up thirty years later you are running from morning to night helping others. You may be doing wonderful things, but you really want to be writing. Your fear of not being a good writer is so deep that you don't even know the wish exists anymore. And you can't acknowledge that you're afraid; that if you stop helping people, for even one second, you will no longer have any value and you might sink into a deep depression. Your altruistic habit is now sucking your real life out of you, but fear of failure at trying anything else keeps you from seeing the truth.

Anxious Times

Unlike our primitive ancestors, contemporary people grow up in an atmosphere of tension. I'm not saying that living in a cave with no personal hygiene or central heating is preferable. But the human organism evolved over millions of years with a nervous system designed to hunt, gather, play, eat, and rest, not necessarily in that order. Fear was programmed in to help the organism escape from a predator, or get shelter from the elements. Children were not torn from their mothers and fed with bottles by nannies, or forced into early toilet training. There were no entrance exams for nursery school. No one ever had to worry about getting fired, or not having the latest blinking-light running shoes, or belonging to the wrong gym, or getting creamed on the highway. There were no taxes; as a matter of fact, there was no money. The first banks weren't created until the Middle Ages! No one drove to work. There weren't even any clocks.

Now, from the minute we are born, anxiety looms everywhere—from the birth room to the boardroom. There is evidence that being denied the nipple, or contact with the mother, is anxiety provoking. According to Joseph Chilton Pearce, world-renowned educator and author of classics in child development like *Magical Child,* contemporary infant rearing actually increases a child's stress level, programming the brain stem, also known as the reptile brain, to be prepared for danger at all times. This constant firing of the fight-or-flight impulse programmed so brilliantly by Mother Nature exhausts the sympathetic nervous system, destroying our immune system and diminishing our potential. A half-hour highway commute triggers the fight-or-flight response more times than a week on the savannah. Instead of enjoying life, and having an occasional adrenaline rush in the face of real danger, our bodies live in a state of constant readiness for the worst. On top of that, the media tries to titillate that very part, leaving us even more frightened—of guns, rapists, fires, mosquitoes, anthrax. The world of entertainment, from violent video games to Armageddon movies, also goes for that same terror response.

People labeled counterphobics try to physically address this by engaging in high-adrenaline activities that exhaust the body and leave them in a state of relaxation afterward—bungee jumping, white-water rafting, surfing, extreme rock climbing come to mind. Others create emotional dramas or choose careers that lead to emotionally draining confrontations—abusive spouses, cheating lovers, political extremists are just a few. Foreign correspondents, firefighters, lion tamers thrive on the adrenaline rush, often at the expense of their personal lives. Whether it's rage or terror, a huge emotional outburst drains the body and releases the tension stored from daily stress.

So you get so used to constant fear, it forms the background of your emotional state. There's always a little voice saying:

"Watch out, that's not good for you."
"Just try that and you'll get hurt!"
"If you do that everyone will laugh at you."
"Don't you dare!"

The body, always being programmed by how you receive stimuli, assumes this is the way you want things. This is what is necessary to survive in this world. So when you want to try something different, make the big leap, walk away, your body literally will not allow you to because the fear program is so strong. Your body actually thinks it's helping you. After all, what if you tell your boss what you really want and she fires you? What if you tell your husband you want to go back to school and he throws you out? What if you decide to open that business and you lose all your money? What if, what if . . . No wonder our shoulders are perpetually hunched up in anticipation of the next disaster!

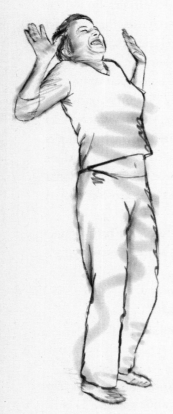

The Startle Reflex

Speaking of shoulders to the ears, many people carry the posture of fear in every step. Some have rounded shoulders, the chest caved in, the neck either protruding forward or the head hanging down. Others have their shoulders pinned back, a perpetually startled look on their faces, eyes darting about, their gestures fast and furtive. Often, one finds variations or combinations of these two extremes.

Both manifestations are again

Illustration 1.1

the result of the innate fear of

falling. If the human baby
senses that it is falling, the first
instinct is shock (*see* illustration
1.1). Then, in order to protect
the viscera, the body curls up
(*see* illustration 1.2). In animals,
this same instinct is triggered
in moments of severe danger. If
the animal is wounded, or overwhelmed by a stronger adversary,
it curls up around its viscera and
plays dead, holding its breath, hop-
ing to protect itself a little longer,
or even fool the assailant. You can
observe this phenomenon in its extreme by visiting a veterans' hospital, where there are soldiers locked
permanently in variations of the startle reflex.

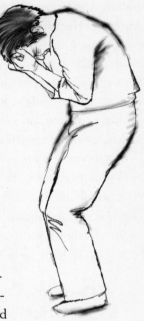

Illustration 1.2

Each present experience, and each future experience you
anticipate, is recorded in your posture, or "acture," as
Feldenkrais called our body language. A perceived childhood trauma, an illness, or an accident may have triggered a
startle reflex response in you. Often, this becomes a habitual
posture that affects every interaction. Interestingly enough,
the chosen posture often physiologically helps reinforce the
fear. For example, when a person's posture is round-shouldered,
the ribs exert a constant pressure on the viscera, effectively
inhibiting proper functioning. Behind the ribs is the solar

plexus, the largest concentration of nerves in the body, also known as the ganglion. When a person is punched in the solar plexus, some bodily functions can actually shut down. And constant pressure downward can also affect this ganglion. In addition, when the spine is rounded, quick turning and use of the arms is more difficult. All of these problems with posture conspire to make the individual weak and unstable, creating more fear!

But it's true that our daily regimen can also affect posture—sitting at a desk all day, for example, often leads to rounded shoulders; ballet dancers can experience overly rotated hips from constantly pointing their feet outward. Most postural habits are the result of stored tension, or "excessive tonus," in specific areas.

→ *Checking Out Your Tension Spots*

Stand quietly with your eyes closed. Imagine a line going down the center of your body. Where is your head in relation to that line? Is your neck in front or behind the line? What about your shoulders? Sometimes one shoulder is in front and one is behind. Is your chest thrust forward of the line, or somewhere behind it? Where is your pelvis? Is your lower back arched? Are your knees relaxed or are they locked? Do you feel the weight on your feet in the middle, front, or back? Perhaps you feel more weight on the left or the right. In an organized body, everything lines up.

If you are unaccustomed to sensing your body, you may not be able to tell. After all, you've lived with this posture your entire life. In that case, look at your profile in a mirror, or have a friend tell you what she sees. Then try again to "sense" what the visual observation is telling you.

Chances are that if you feel yourself "out of line," you are using tension to hold yourself in place. Take a fresh stance. Now notice: Are you really comfortable?

The Difficult Question

You can become so accustomed to being uncomfortable that you no longer feel tension or pain. But if you practice checking out your tension spots, you'll begin to notice discomfort in the background, coloring your mood and your thoughts. It is the body's response to stress. You may want to try surveying yourself at different times—working at your desk, cooking, even while talking to someone. Once you've determined that there is indeed tension in how you sit, how you chop onions, how you hold the phone to your ear, you need to ask yourself: Why am I tense? Am I afraid of something?

Fear defeats more people than any other one thing in the world.   — RALPH WALDO EMERSON

2. Symptoms of Fear

We have many clever strategies for coping with our fear. Our society has become so acclimated to living in this state of perpetual anxiety that some manifestations of fear are actually the cultural norm. Answer the following questions as honestly as possible:

Do people accuse you of being a workaholic?

Are you a procrastinator?

Do you often watch TV instead of other activities?

Do you feel "under the weather" more than once a week?

Do you drink or take recreational drugs more than once or twice a week?

Do you overeat?

Do little things piss you off to no end?

Do you have trouble sleeping?

Do you have trouble getting out of bed?

Do you program your day with an impossibly long "to do" list?

Do you get so caught up in unnecessary details that you never get to certain things on your "to do" list?

Do you resent others' success?

Do you sometimes feel paralyzed?

Do you cry a lot over your situation?

Does life feel boring?

Do you feel like there's never time to do what you truly wish?

If you answered yes to two or more of these questions, fear is in your life.

Fear has many disguises. It can pose as depression: it's just impossible to get excited over anything; just clearing the debris off of your desk seems titanic, let alone buying the newspaper and looking at the want ads. And, of course, depression can masquerade as tiredness. You're so exhausted; how could you possibly go to that swing dance club, or even the gym, where you might—just might—encounter someone destined to be your partner? Or you feel sick. People have reported literally feeling like they might puke if they had to make "the phone call," whether it was to tell Mom that, no, I'm not coming this weekend, to or make an appointment at an art gallery to show artwork. We've all heard stories of actors vomiting before they went on stage. But they *do* go on the stage. What is the difference between the trapeze artist running to the bathroom and then leaping into the void and the person who uses the symptoms of sickness to keep from leaping into life?

It's the payoff. The skydiver trusts that sometime after jumping out of the plane there's going to be a moment of suspension in another dimension, an opportunity to feel like a bird, and the rush of landing safely. The performer gets to share her experience, plus receive validation in the form of applause. For each of them, the payoff is more valuable than comfort. But when you're paralyzed by fear, the payoff seems slim, or nonexistent.

Let's say you tried to free yourself from your mother before. You defied her wishes, and instead of going for a nursing degree you went for a degree in anthropology. You couldn't get a job anywhere after graduation and ended up having to learn computer programming, which you hate, just to pay the bills. The boyfriend she despised all along ditched you. Now it's less painful to just spend time with her than to break away from her power. She's obviously right: You *are* a loser!

Or perhaps your dad was the most amazing man ever. Whatever you needed always magically appeared. He could fix anything. You never had to lift a finger, in fact, because Dad always did whatever needed doing so much better than you. He even got you that first job when you got out of college. Sure, you thought about being an illustrator, but you owe Dad so much you'd never tell him you prefer working in the arts rather than insurance, let alone tell him you're gay and break his heart.

When all you can see is a negative outcome, or you fear the price is greater than the reward, your body will stop you from moving. Literally. That's why some people work at a job they hate for twenty to thirty years, then die of a heart attack.

Counterphobia

There is a term in psychology called counterphobia; that is, when a person engages in an activity other people consider risky in order to hide his own fear. Many an actor will confess that she is terribly shy. A person afraid of seeming inadequate might become a bodybuilder, maybe even a politician. Often the strategy is so successful that the individual no longer senses the underlying fear that motivated the original choice.

"It's a mystery," replied the Lion. "I suppose I was born that way. All the other animals in the forest naturally expect me to be brave, for the Lion is everywhere thought to be the King of Beasts. I learned that if I roared very loudly every living thing was frightened and got out of my way. Whenever I've met a man I've been awfully scared; but I just roared at him, and he has always run away as fast as he could go. If the elephants and the tigers and the bears had ever tried to fight me, I should have run myself—I'm such a coward; but just as soon as they

hear me roar they all try to get away from me, and of
course I let them go."

—L. FRANK BAUM, *The Wonderful Wizard of Oz*

These people are often very high functioning, and you
could *never* imagine accusing them of being afraid. Yet, by
disguising their terror, even if unconsciously, they are causing stress to their system. If the fear is not recognized and
acknowledged, it can lead to unexplainable pain, disease,
and anxiety disorders.

Dietrich is a brilliant and highly successful writer. He
grew up in a violently dysfunctional household where
abuse came often and unexpectedly. Chasing chaos, he
ended up as a political reporter for a major daily newspaper.
Describing himself as "an adrenaline junkie," Dietrich
risked life and limb to uncover sordid tales of political
corruption and to scoop other reporters in undercover in-
vestigative coups. He worked late and frantic hours in order to drown the unexplainable sense of terror and dread
that dogged him. Finally, in a state of utter exhaustion,
his body began to fall apart. His shoulders froze, his fingers became paralyzed, and he was diagnosed with carpal
tunnel syndrome. Dietrich had to stop writing and begin
to take care of himself.

After a few lessons in the Feldenkrais Method, which
helped him see the connection between his terror and his
pain, Dietrich began attending yoga classes. The quiet

meditation and relaxation sequences were the first time he had allowed rest into his life in over twenty years. Often tears rose unbidden, without words, without logic, yet afterward he felt better. While not able to quite forgive his parents, he was able to let go of their grip on his psyche. He quit his job and is now working freelance. Sometimes, he takes on too many assignments; he can feel that frantic adrenaline-laced tension once again mounting in his shoulders, and he realizes that some kind of anxiety is looking for recognition. That's when he puts the client on hold, canceling the job or passing it on to a colleague, and heads over to the yoga studio.

The First Step

Acknowledging that you are afraid is the first step. It's one thing to know you're afraid and pretend that you're not in order to forge ahead; it's quite another to be so far away from yourself that you don't even know that fear is motivating your action/inaction. Before you can even begin to uncover *what* you are afraid of, you need to admit fear exists. The following exercises can help you begin to verify for yourself whether you live in the grip of fear or not. Many times, lying to yourself only blocks the sound of the howling wolves in your consciousness. So listen carefully to your responses. If you consistently say you feel nothing, or you feel angry and outraged at the exercise/question, it's possible that you are in deep denial.

Andrea signed up for my workshop way in advance, happily sending me a check with a long note about how important my work would be for society. She explained that she had evolved out of fear long ago through years of work on herself and that now she was only occasionally startled by a loud noise or a bug landing on her. The first night of the workshop as people introduced themselves and why they came, she launched into a lengthy monologue about her lack of fear and how she came here merely to understand better this phenomenon that seems to plague humans. At the end of the evening, I was having difficulty with a door and called for someone to give a pull on the other side. A man she was speaking to leaped up to help me. We chatted for a few minutes and went back inside. Andrea was sulking in the corner. That night, she e-mailed to say she could not attend the rest of the workshop, that she could not possibly trust a group of people that would be so willing to abandon her in the middle of a conversation.

You will need a notebook. It can be something you already write in, or you may want to have a special book just for this work. Don't do these exercises all at once—allow some space between them.

➔ *Beginning to Listen*

Find a quiet space where you can sit comfortably, either on a chair or a cushion. In order to be truly free of constraints, you can bring in an alarm clock set to go off in twenty minutes. That way, you won't have to keep looking at the clock—and, believe me, you'll want to. Sit with your eyes closed and begin to listen to your breathing. Just notice: How do you breathe? Try to keep your attention on your breath. You will drift off. Each time you return, come back to sensing your breath, but note what was on your mind as you drifted away. Were you replaying a conversation? Planning tomorrow's agenda? Singing a song from your youth? Don't judge, just notice. You can even say to yourself, "I'm thinking about the fight I had with Jeff," or, "I'm planning my shopping trip." Then let it go.

At the end of the twenty minutes, take your notebook, jot down the places you went to, the thoughts that came to you, the emotions that went through you, even if they seem dumb right now.

Do this exercise at least six times, either once a day, or spread out over the week as it works in your schedule. After doing the exercise six times, take a look at what you have written. Notice if you went to the same or different places each time. Were your thoughts mostly in the future or the past? Are there emotions associated with any of the thoughts that came up? How many of them are "negative"? What did the pleasant daydreams or fantasies dwell on? How often did you go off in a repetitive song, or just counting? That is a strategy of the mind/body to keep you from feeling something.

There are several exercises in this book that invite you to explore the state of your mind/body system. Although the nature of a book requires that the instructions be read, you have other options for experiencing these somatic explorations. If you prefer, you can read these exercises out loud into a recorder, then play them back, following the verbal instructions. You can have a friend read the instructions as you execute them. Alternatively, you can log on to www.laviniaplonka.com and download free audio versions of these lessons as you need them. The exercises that are available online are marked with an icon (⟩).

→ *Listening to the Body* ⟩

Lie on your back, either on a carpet or a mat. If you need a pillow or something under your head or legs, arrange things to make it comfortable. Notice the parts of yourself that easily contact the floor. Sense the quality of your breathing. Feel your back, your shoulders, your buttocks, your hands. Now let your thoughts drift a little bit, until you encounter a thought, image, or picture that involves some kind of personal difficulty. It could be a family situation, a career issue, an unfinished project, a panicky situation. Now take the time to see all the details surrounding the issue. See the environment, the person's face (if there is a person involved). Play out the conversation; start to *sense* what's going on. As you do this, let your attention travel to your body. Has it changed? Where do you feel a difference? Wherever you feel tension residing, ask yourself if this is a familiar feeling, almost comfortable in its discomfort. Notice your breathing. Is this familiar as well? Can you relate any of this experience of yourself to the startle reflex mentioned earlier?

Now choose something that you noticed. Perhaps it was a tightening in the belly. Or clenching your jaw. Maybe your toes curled. For a few moments, intentionally exaggerate what you noticed. If you were hunching your shoulders, hunch them more. Stay there and try to keep breathing for around ten seconds. Then, slowly, let that part go. You can repeat this for as many places you noticed.

Often, in the beginning, people say they notice nothing. Be patient with yourself. It is not part of our culture to notice the body, so beginning to sense yourself is like learning a new language. And sometimes, something in you doesn't want to sense. If you sense what's going on, all hell might break loose! Honor your body's intelligence, take your time, and trust the process.

There's nothing wrong with being afraid. H. P. Lovecraft once said, "Fear is the oldest and strongest emotion of mankind." Power comes from admitting fear and then having the courage to try anyway. Paralyzing fear really is parasitic, sapping energy, robbing you of your full potential. In denying the existence of fear, you are living a lie. In "The Tell-Tale Heart," Edgar Allan Poe's protagonist goes mad with the fear of being discovered as a murderer. He is so desperate to hide the terror he feels that he actually hears the heart of the man he murdered beating underneath the floor where he hid the body. When I was a child, it was always a kind of relief to get caught, to finally admit to my pecadillo or lie. The stress of lying to *yourself* is even greater. The old cliché "You can run but you can't hide" is especially true when running from yourself. Taking the time to discover and *name* what you're feeling is essential in moving toward a courageous life.

3. *So, What Are You Afraid Of?*

cknowledging that fear exists is a powerful first step. Discovering the *source* of your inner trembling can be like searching for the Holy Grail. The truth is, the answer is right there in front of you, but you yourself get in your own way. In one version of the legend of the Holy Grail, the hero Parsifal comes to the palace guarding the Holy Grail. All kinds of strange and wondrous things are presented to him, including a wounded king. He's a marvelous king, but obviously suffering tremendously from his wound. Parsifal is embarrassed and talks about everything else except what is so obvious, that the king is seriously wounded. His mentor had always told him that good knights don't ask too many questions, so he keeps his mouth shut. Meanwhile, the secret to saving the suffering king and winning the Holy Grail was to dare to ask the king, "Of what wound are you suffering?" It just never occurred to Parsifal to actually ask what he was thinking.

Looking for the source of fear sometimes invites difficult questions, questions that themselves evoke fear. It's only natural to want to stay comfortable, continuing along the same old path. It may be miserable, but it's a familiar misery that doesn't force you to look at the gaping wound right in front of your face.

Blind Spots

A very common nightmare is being chased. People often report that they don't know what or who is chasing them, and usually they wake up screaming, trembling, or in some other state of high anxiety. Professionals often recommend that in these dreams one should stop, turn around, and confront the attacker. Supposedly, by facing the fear, and identifying it, you regain power. Now, this seems like a lovely idea. And there may be people out there who can control their dreams. But most of us are pretty powerless in our sleep. Sometimes we even dream that we're *awake,* talking about the dream we had, only to wake up and realize, Wait a second, that was a dream too! I believe when you *are ready* to confront your assailant in your dream, then you are able to turn around. And it's the same thing in our waking life.

There are many traditions that call this "waking life" a dream as well. The Hindus call our existence Maya, saying that, somewhere, Vishnu is napping and we are his dream. Toltec and Yaqui Indian traditions both call our ordinary

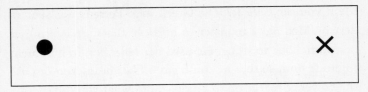

Illustration 3.1

waking life dreaming. The blockbuster movie *The Matrix* suggests that we are all just part of a huge computer program. We have the illusion of control because we feel solid, and things happen sort of logically. But just as in our sleeping dreams, there are things we cannot control or see.

Try the following experiment. Hold this book up so that the illustration (*see* illustration 3.1) is at arm's length, in front of both your eyes. Close your left eye, and focus the right eye on the dark circle. Keeping your left eye closed, slowly bring the book closer to your face. Between ten to fourteen inches from your nose, the X in the box should disappear. This is what is known as your vision's blind spot, the area on your retina where the optic nerve passes through and therefore leaves your eye "blind" to any images that fall there.

Just as your eyes can't see at a certain angle, the thing you fear may be just out of the corner of your perception. Medicine calls it a "scotoma," a shadow or block in your perception. Your friends and family can probably see very clearly that you're afraid to leave your job, spouse, old house, but even if they told you you wouldn't hear or understand them. That is the nature of the psychological blind spot.

So how can you turn around and face your fear in waking

life if you can't see it? The Greek hero Perseus was sent to destroy Medusa, a monster so horrible that just looking at her turned one to stone. He used her reflection in his shield to guide him, so that he could cut off her head. You can use the power of reflection to guide you to what you can't see.

→ The Mirror

Imagine that your emotions and reactions are a mirror of your fear. The things that make you feel happy and excited speak to your confident side. When you become whiny, negative, irritated, angry—take these reactions as alarm bells. Something around this person, task, situation is stirring up fear. Begin to notice those moments, and then when the opportunity arises ask yourself: What am I afraid of? Write what comes up in your notebook.

→ Reflection/Recapitulation

Many times things happen so fast, it's often impossible to remember to try the above exercise, or to keep track of what's happening. That's why it's useful before you go to bed at night to sit quietly or lie down on a carpet or mat. Close your eyes and begin to replay your day in reverse. Notice what happens. As you reflect on a difficult moment, sense the change in your breathing, your muscle "tonus." Are there sections of the day you want to skip over? They're exactly the ones to examine! Are there points in the playback when you suddenly space out and drift away, only to come back a few moments later, not remembering how you got to that thought? This is the body trying to shield you from a blind spot. In the beginning, it will be difficult to remember much. But then things pop up the next day. And as you become more courageous, you will literally see more.

Sometimes, we have no trouble naming fears. I'm afraid of the dark. I'm afraid to go outside. I'm afraid to ask my boss for a raise. Yet all of these fears may be distractions, disguises for what's lurking in your blind spot.

"I must not fear. Fear is the mind-killer. Fear is the little-death that brings total obliteration. I will face my fear. I will permit it to pass over me and through me. And when it has gone past I will turn the inner eye to see its path. Where the fear has gone there will be nothing. Only I will remain."   —"Litany Against Fear," from the novel *Dune* by FRANK HERBERT

Symptoms vs. Causes

You know those little Russian nesting dolls called matrioshkas? It's a wooden doll, and, when you open it, inside is a smaller doll identical to the first. And then when you open the smaller doll you discover yet another, even smaller doll, and so on until you get to a teeny little replica of the first doll.

Uncovering the cause of fear can be like that, only in reverse. Many people live their lives built on excuses: I hate parties; I'm afraid to go out; I get panic attacks; I'm tired. All of these are like a bunch of little dolls hiding the *giant* doll, the core of fear.

As was said earlier, we are born with one instinctive fear—fear of falling. This fear, of course, is connected with the primal fear: the fear of death. Since all creatures' prime directive is survival, often this core fear develops in childhood, when we feel helpless and vulnerable. Children quickly learn to fear illness, starvation, abandonment. Because, after all, the result of any of those is—you got it—death.

Now, of course, it seems ridiculous, growing up in a happy, middle-class family, or even in an unhappy, struggling family, for a four-year-old to worry about starvation. But they do, although it's often unconscious. They quietly develop survival strategies even the most loving parents wouldn't dream of. They learn to be aggressive, to protect themselves. Or they become supernice, always staying out of the way, trying not to take up too much space. Or maybe they turn into overachievers, trying to prove their worth. Somewhere along the line, the chosen survival strategy becomes habit. The fear of starvation, abandonment—whatever—disappears from memory, and all that's left is a gnawing anxiety every time the grown-up child tries to deviate from the pattern developed many years before.

Of course, not everyone grew up in a perfect home. Real trauma can lead to all kinds of fears in adult life. Abusive parents, a devastating illness, the unexpected death of a loved one—many events can create an indelible impression that affects the rest of your life. Sometimes children create imagined traumas that lie buried beneath their adult selves, unaware that a misinterpreted memory is sabotaging their happiness.

When Melody was two years old, her parents, burned-out from overwork, decided to take a three-day weekend, leaving her with her grandmother. She had never been away from her parents for more than a few hours, and even those few hours often left her in tears. Mommy and Daddy explained that they would be gone a few days, but Melody didn't really understand what a few days were. Minutes stretched into hours, into days. She wailed inconsolably. Each time a car drove by, she hurled herself at the door. By the third day, exhausted, she sat staring into space. When her happy and relaxed parents returned, Melody just stared at them. She didn't speak for two weeks. Her parents were beside themselves. Slowly, Melody resumed communication. Even though as Melody got older she forgot the event, each time they left the house she suffered an unexplainable anxiety attack. As an adult, she lived in constant fear of abandonment—by her friends, her husband, her children—without knowing why. In therapy, she relived a memory of her parents abandoning her alone in an empty house. When she confronted them, they told her the above story, trying to set things straight. But knowing the truth did not help Melody relax. Her body still feared the abandonment! Eventually, through work with her physical reactions and using breathing to ground her, Melody was able to let go of this imagined trauma and live a fuller life.

Whether the trauma is real or imagined, remembered or forgotten becomes irrelevant when you decide to address your current fears. All the investigating and intellectualizing in the world will not alter the program you've had running in your mind/body system because there has been a physiological change to your brain. Psychology calls this manifestation post-traumatic stress disorder, or PTSD. For the last several years, a lot of research has gone into trying to figure out whether stress and trauma actually affect the body. Much evidence points to an actual brain change due to stress. According to J. Douglas Bremner of the Yale Psychiatric Institute, stress hormones, called glucocortisoids, affect the hippocampus and perhaps other parts of the brain. According to the National Center for PTSD, the hippocampus plays an important part in how our memories are formed and stored. Through magnetic resonance imaging (what we call an MRI), it has been shown that the hippocampi of people who suffer from post-traumatic stress disorder are actually altered. Short-term memory is damaged; new learning possibilities have been compromised. In spite of its best efforts, the brain's tape recorder just keeps on replaying the past over and over, like a loop.

The only way to change the program is to reorganize the mind/body system. Although there isn't definitive proof that the brain damage can be reversed, there have been success stories among people suffering from PTSD through cognitive therapy; that is, learning new habits. And studies have shown that the hippocampus can actually regenerate neurons. One of the best ways to improve the function of the nervous system is to learn; one of the best ways to learn is to take time to be with yourself.

The following exercises are not intended for you to recall or analyze past events. You may or may not discover the initial causes of your fears. However, you will come closer, hopefully, to seeing how these fears affect every aspect of your life now, and, from there, you can begin to take more concrete action.

→ *Unresolved Issues*

Sit down with your notebook or a sheet of paper. Make two columns. Head the first column "Issues," the second column "What am I afraid of?" Then let your mind wander for a few minutes. Without thinking too much, in the first column quickly list five unfinished/unresolved issues hanging over you. For example: call about selling the car; talk to Mom re: Dad's clothes to Goodwill; pay the electric bill; sort drawers; settle argument with Jerry. Under the second column, What am I afraid of?, write down the fear that pops up next to each issue. Your mind may balk at this; after all, why should I be afraid of calling about the car? Certainly I'm not afraid to pay the electric bill! Even if it seems silly, just allow whatever fear appears in your mind to sit right next to the task. If absolutely nothing comes up, let it go, your mind will eventually wander back to it. Now you may have a list that looks like this:

ISSUES	WHAT AM I AFRAID OF?
Call about selling the car	Afraid no one will buy it
Mom re: Dad's clothes to Goodwill	Afraid she'll freak out
Pay the electric bill	Afraid I can't pay the rent
Sort drawers	Afraid I'm wasting time
Confront Jerry	Afraid he won't listen

Such apparently minor issues can really show you your deeper fears. Afraid no one will buy your car? Does that mean your car is worthless, and therefore so are you? Or are you afraid no one will buy it and therefore you won't be able to afford your new car and you'll lose your car, your house, your wife . . . Our fears seem silly to the intellectual mind, but they still remain locked in our bodies unless we listen to the deeper questions rocking around inside each event. If Mom freaks out, will she not love you anymore? You know intellectually, of course, that that's not true, but your childhood fear of rejection by a parental figure keeps you from dealing with something apparently small.

Even though the fear you put beside each issue seems small, if you dig deep enough you will see that it connects to some anxiety about survival—rejection, starvation, harm. Try it for yourself.

Peeling the Layers

Phrases such as "I don't like" or "It's boring" protect you from uncomfortable feelings. They are so effective, often you can't find anything else underneath the sense that something is annoying or pisses you off. But as was said earlier, sadness and anger are surefire signs that fear is hiding underneath. That is not to say that by admitting your fear, you have to start doing the thing you fear. Just because you are afraid to ride horses doesn't mean you have to force yourself to do it. But looking at the feelings surrounding horseback riding, for example, can help you see many other related emotions that may be stopping you in other aspects of your life. And maybe you can come to embrace that activity as well.

I was around twenty-two years old, not a great swimmer, but always wanting to prove how cool I was. My younger sister just *was* cool. We were in Cozumel where we met several handsome, articulate men who were expert scuba divers. They offered to teach us. I wanted to go on the boat. I wanted to be around the men. My sister seemed to genuinely want to dive. But I didn't really want to go in the water. After all, how great could it be, just flapping around looking at the same fish you can see at the aquarium, dragging all that equipment on your back, breathing through your mouth, fogging up your mask. It seemed more trouble than it was worth. But I was too proud to be outdone by my sister.

They took us to a pond, dressed us up in the gear, and

we dove. I couldn't breathe. Sitting on the bottom of the pond, I took huge gulps of air from my regulator, but there was no air. I felt as if I was about to explode. I signaled my ascent and shot to the surface. I tore the regulator from my mouth and gasped. One of the guys came up and asked what was wrong. Still hyperventilating, I pointed to the regulator. "It's not working!" I managed to choke out. "I'm getting out!" He came over to me and held my shoulders. He clamped the regulator on my mouth and held my nose. "Breathe in!" he commanded. I did. "Breathe out!" Amazingly, air was coming in and going out of my lungs. He smiled compassionately. "Fear is incredibly powerful, isn't it?" he asked.

Later, as I darted through the water, buoyant and graceful among the dazzling corals, anemones, and schools of angelfish, I marveled that I could have denied myself such an experience simply by not acknowledging my fear of drowning.

→ I Just Don't Like It

In one column, list five things you don't like to do; for example, go to parties, exercise, do bills, drive, ride a horse. In a second column, write down the way these things make you *feel*. For example: Exercise—Is boring and too difficult. Then make a third column and head it: What am I afraid of? This is the hard part. Could it be that you find exercise boring because you're afraid to get into it? Is it too difficult because you chose a program that's too hard for you, so that you're destined for failure? There are many reasons why you "don't like" something. Now it's time to dig, suspend judgment, and be sincere. If nothing comes up, that's okay; you'll see it eventually. Just move on.

It's possible that you will experience a paradox: the fear of uncovering your fear. You are an intricately designed system that has somehow managed to survive, even thrive, with the postures and behavior patterns developed over a lifetime. Your body *wants* to keep things as they are. Remember, even if it's miserable it's safe. If you should start digging around, you might want to change things, and change spells instability. If you find yourself experiencing fear, anger, or other difficult emotions as you do the above exercises, pause, take a breath. Talk to someone, write what's going on, go for a swim, change your angle of inquiry. Don't push it. Don't run away. Otherwise, the truth will not reveal itself. Trust the process.

Part II

Facing Your Fear

4. Fear of Injury or Death

We all want to protect ourselves from illness and injury. No one wants to die prematurely, or be debilitated and dependent. Avoiding pain, taking care of your health, not engaging in foolhardy activities are all sensible ways to live longer.

Sometimes, however, this self-protective mechanism takes precedence over enjoying life. The irony is that it often seems the more afraid you are that something is going to happen, the more likely it is that something will happen! Anxiety and obsessing about illness can actually depress the immune system, making you more susceptible to the very thing you are afraid of.

One way this happens is the result of the fight-or-flight response already discussed. In true danger, the response is triggered, sending cortisol and adrenaline coursing through your system. These stressors are known to cause tissue breakdown. Once a real emergency is over, the body stops producing these chemicals. But when stress and worry are constantly present, the neurons just keep firing, the chemicals keep on entering the system, eventually compromising health. In a *Tampa Tribune* article, Charles D. Spielberger, a psychology professor at the University of South Florida and president-elect of the American Psychological Association, has stated, "Your mood influences your immune system. You can wear it out. It can affect your susceptibility to colds, and in the long term even to cancer and other diseases."

Conversely, there have been many studies that correlate a positive attitude with healing. One of the most famous was done at Stanford University. For one year, eighty-six women with metastatic breast cancer took part in group therapy sessions where they were encouraged to share their experiences and form bonds with the other women. In a follow-up study ten years later, the researchers found that the women who participated in the psychosocial interventions lived an average of two years longer than those who did not. The researchers were amazed, since their intention was to prove the opposite. "We intended, in particular, to examine the often overstated claims made by those who teach cancer patients that the right mental attitude will help to conquer the disease."*

---

*David Spiegel, "Effect of psychosocial treatment on survival of patients with metastatic breast cancer," *Lancet* 2 (8668): 888–91.

Another way that fear of injury or pain can create a "self-fulfilling prophecy" is how your performance level is affected under duress. Nervousness about, say, having a car accident can make the body so tense, you are more prone to be a dangerous driver, putting yourself at risk of an accident. Sometimes, the fear can completely paralyze you, making life not worth living.

Pain and Suffering

Pain is a very important neurological message. If you felt no pain when you broke your leg, you'd continue to walk on it and destroy it. If you felt no pain with a stomach ulcer, your entire digestive system could collapse. Norman Cousins, in his book *Anatomy of an Illness,* speaks about Dr. Brand, a surgeon who studied lepers. When a leprous boy successfully turned a key in a rusty lock that Dr. Brand had been unable to open, "[h]e examined the boy's thumb and forefinger of the right hand. The key had cut the flesh to the bone. The boy had been completely unaware of what was happening to his fingers while turning the key. . . . The desensitized nerve endings had made it possible for the hand to keep turning the key long past the point where a healthy person would have found it painful to continue."

This is one extreme. A healthy person can generally recognize when pain is just sore muscles, or an indication that something should be checked out. But for some, even the slightest pain sends their internal program to instant tragedy—"Something is terribly wrong with me!"—initiating fear of death. For others, avoiding pain becomes almost an obsession. If you have had an injury, for example, even something minor like a cut finger, suddenly all movement, all activities, are centered around protecting that finger. When there is a more serious injury, or a chronic pain illness such as fibromyalgia, life becomes a dance of avoidance and limitation as the fear of pain dominates all life choices. Fear of pain can become a force that controls every move, every activity, even if that pain is not connected to tissue damage.

Obsessing and Worrying

Tom used illness to get attention when he was little—perfectly understandable with dysfunctional parents who basically ignored the children unless something was wrong. He was constantly getting sent home from school with a stomachache, which irritated his stressed-out, carless mother no end because she had to call neighbors to pick him up or get her husband to leave work. One day, he began to experience severe stomach pains. His teacher felt this was yet another gambit for attention and made him stay at his desk till the end of the day. He got home and fell on the kitchen floor, at which point his mother sent him to his room until he "got over it." When his mother came upstairs, she found him unconscious with blood and bile all over the sheets. Tom had peritonitis from a burst appendix. It took him months to recover. His shaken parents waited on him hand and foot. Each time Tom felt a pain, or unwell, the whole household went into a panic.

As an adult, Tom couldn't shake the feeling that everything was a deadly disease. His hand would tremble slightly and he was instantly in the medical encyclopedia, combing the Internet, convinced he had Lou Gehrig's disease. Moles were melanoma. Headaches were an aneurysm. It seems laughable, but it was the bane of Tom's life.

Tom's system, after this trauma, had decided that any symptom was a cause for "red alert." This was a survival strategy. The other, hidden factor was his need for attention. His mind/body system still craved the unconditional love, the nurturing that had replaced his family's regular chaos as they nursed him through convalescence.

Tom slowly began to recognize triggers that set off his "I'm dying" program. He noticed that it happened when things were either going really badly, or really well. He could eventually trace both to fear. When life became stressful and he was afraid he couldn't cope, a physical symptom became cause for alarm. Ironically, when things were going too well he also experienced the same panic. It was related to his belief that he did not deserve happiness; therefore, something horrible had to happen. He now uses these moments of fear as reminders to relax, take some time for himself and his body.

"I'm very brave generally," he went on in a low voice: "only today I happen to have a headache."

—LEWIS CARROLL, *Through the Looking Glass*

It is important to differentiate when pain is a signal for medical attention, and when it is trying to keep you from living your life. The pain itself is sometimes your mind/body system trying to keep you from doing what you fear! It's really easy to get out of going to a party where you might have to interact with people who intimidate you because you have a headache. Or to not go for a walk that might help you lose weight because you have lower back pain. Your lower back pain, in fact, might be the result of your inactivity and weight gain. Many books have been written about this. However, for the purposes of our study here, let's look at three mind/body ways to work with pain and illness and their relationship to fear.

➔ The Body Landscape

Take a sheet of paper and pencil and draw a picture of your body—a stick figure, an outline, an abstract interpretation; it doesn't matter. It's just for you, and you'll be referring back to it throughout this exercise. Now, mark the areas that bother you: maybe it's a specific pain; maybe it's some part of you you know is damaged already; maybe it's just a part of you you just don't like, like your hips are too wide, for example. Use color pencils to circle or darken those areas—and have fun with it! If you wish, label areas with what worries you: maybe this ache is arthritis, or that knee needs surgery, or could this feeling mean liver cancer, and so on.

Now put the drawing aside and lie down comfortably on the floor. Close your eyes and pretend that you have "inner vision" that can scan your body from the inside. Starting with your toes, slowly begin to let these "inner eyes" move upward. Notice if there are areas that are easier to "see" than others. Don't judge or evaluate, just notice.

Once you have gone from toes to the head, just rest.

Now slowly and gently begin rolling your right leg inward and outward. Make it the smallest possible movement that still includes everything from the hip joint down to the foot. Very softly, roll the leg so that you become a little pigeon-toed, and then a little turned out. As you roll your leg, notice your breath. See if you can breathe softly and regularly. If it's not possible, note when you hold your breath.

Rest.

Were there any parts of your leg that were difficult to sense when you scanned in the beginning? Are you able to sense them now, or not?

Notice what you are thinking. After about thirty seconds, try the same thing with the left leg. Try the same thing with your head. Gently roll it from side to side. How small of a movement can you do and still feel you are rolling? How far down your spine can you feel the rolling action? Can you feel your spine at all?

Rest again.

Continue to explore yourself in this way—with your

arms, your pelvis, your chest. These movements should be tiny. It's possible that someone coming into the room and observing you on the floor might not see movement at all.

After spending some time with yourself in this way, repeat the scan that you did in the beginning. Just let your inner eyes travel up and down your body softly, noting areas that perhaps are still unclear. Maybe some areas have surfaced. Are there areas that seem more relaxed, more comfortable? Just lie there, relaxing, and sense your breathing. See if you can tune in to a slight sensation in the back of your head. As if there was a little buzz of conversation happening just beyond your actual comprehension. Softly, without straining, just listen. The first few times you may hear absolutely nothing. It's normal; our minds are programmed to ignore our background states. Yet these inner voices are what create our perceptions.

Antonio Damasio describes what he calls background feelings: "A background feeling corresponds . . . to the body state prevailing *between* emotions. When we feel happiness, anger, or another emotion, the background feeling has been superseded by an emotional feeling. The background feeling is our image of the body landscape when it is not shaken by emotion."

You may actually experience a feeling—tension, or sadness. It may come as words—"You're not good enough," "Hurry!," "I can't." Just lie there, breathe, and listen. Notice if your body gets tense anywhere.

Now, let all this effort you focused on scanning go away. Gently bend your knees and bring your feet to standing. Very softly, let your knees move left and right. If you have back pain, be especially gentle. If you want to feel a little invigorated, let your knees tilt slowly to each side as far as you wish, feeling your whole spine respond.

Rest.

After you rest, go back to your drawing and take a look at it. It's a map of your body fears. Is anything different? Clearer? Feel free to make notes and comments on the drawing—"Stomach seems quieter," "Maybe it's not arthritis," "Better check with the doctor on this one"—whatever comes up, without editing. You may want to change some shapes, some colors. You even may have discovered new areas of interest.

For the rest of the day, each time you are seized by that awful feeling that something is terribly wrong, visualize your drawing. Then take a few moments to sense your breath, and to tune in to that background conversation.

You may have noticed in the above exercise that certain thoughts kept coming up. Sometimes they refuse to hide below the surface. We dwell on them, obsess about them. "I can't, just can't, go to the city," we fret. "Every time I go, I get a migraine headache. Just the thought of it makes me sick." Or, "What's that mole? It's cancer. I know it's cancer. It's going to be as bad as when Mom died. I can't bear it. Oh my God!"

There are several ways to look at these conversations. When you're watching a sitcom on television and all of a sudden a voice-over comes on and says "We interrupt this program with a special news bulletin . . ." you instantly forget the sitcom! All you can think is "What happened? Oh boy, am I in danger?" Daily cares and responsibilities go out the window with this powerful piece of information. It owns you. That's the same thing that happens when these parasitic thoughts take over your mind. And it's often impossible to stop them from replaying over and over again in your head. Imagine you were working on a project on your computer and then all of a sudden another program starts running. You may be irritated, but you can't get back to your "regularly scheduled program." Or you may become so interested in it that you forget what you were doing.

Whether these worrisome thoughts are the result of real or imagined trauma, or a lifetime of conditioning—for example, your mother lived in constant fear of disease—they don't have to stop your life. However, trying to push these thoughts away, or living in denial of them, is not the solution. You need to recognize and acknowledge them. These thoughts are your body trying to tell you something: You are afraid. It's not important to analyze the cause or figure things out. In fact, that can sometimes lead to other obsessive thoughts. Instead, you can work in the present, to begin to teach your body alternative ways to respond to these fears.

→ *A Thought Journal*

This exercise will take some time, but you've already spent a lot of time worrying so let's see if a small investment at this point can yield some insight. Take a small notebook or even a sheet of paper that you can carry with you in your pocket or your purse and keep it handy. For about a week, every time you catch yourself obsessing about a potential illness jot down the time, the thought, and what was going on at the time (having your morning coffee, driving to work, arguing with your spouse). Before the thought fades, notice if you can feel any kind of reaction in yourself—a sinking feeling in the pit of your stomach, tension in your shoulders, wanting to cry. It may even be something apparently unconnected, like curling the toes, for example. Of course, if the thoughts occur while you're driving, wait until you've parked the car to write things down.

In a way, you're doing the same thing people do when they see a nutritionist and are asked to write down all the foods they've eaten for the past week. Our thoughts are a kind of food—you can have toxic thoughts and you can have nourishing thoughts. And your system craves the toxic thoughts as much as the nourishing ones, just like a body out of balance craves sugar or alcohol.

Think of yourself as a kind of Sherlock Holmes trying to uncover the culprits. After a week has gone by, take a look at your list. Did thoughts appear randomly? At particular times of day? After a particular activity or encounter? How many times a day did they occur? How long did the thoughts go on before you stopped them or they were interrupted? Were your feelings/sensations the same or different each time? Go back to the drawing of your body that you did in the earlier exercise. Circle or shade in the parts of your body that you noticed during the week. While they don't have to necessarily correspond to your original observations, they might. Just take note of the drawing, as if you are looking at a map of the country you call you.

→ Posture, Tension, and Emotion

Find a comfortable position, either lying down or sitting, and close your eyes. Let your attention softly travel to one of the areas of your body that you noticed during the week. Now intentionally tense that area. Clench, squeeze, or grip your muscles. As you do so, sense your breath. See if you can feel what happens in the rest of yourself. After about fifteen seconds, let it go. Sense yourself again. Is anything different? You can repeat this exercise for all the tension spots you experienced.

It's possible that you didn't notice physical sensations, but maybe you did feel angry, or even like crying. In that case, see if you can create in yourself the posture you have when you are having that emotion. Scrunch your shoulders, grit your teeth—whatever you can remember. Many studies have shown that when people assume a posture evocative of an emotion, they actually start to feel that emotion growing in themselves. Susannah Bloch, a Chilean scientist experimenting with this idea, has developed a new technique for actors based on her research: the Alba Emoting Method. Actors study the posture, facial expressions, and breathing patterns of various emotions and evolve characters out of the physiological experience of the posture. Bloch posits that the physiological changes in posture signal the brain to release the chemicals that result in the emotion. By *intentionally* re-creating the posture, you learn how the emotion arises in you.

By practicing the above exercise a few times during the week, your body/mind system is going to begin to understand how it responds to what it perceives as danger. Then, when you find yourself in your obsessing/worrying mode, you can quickly sense what is physically taking place. At that point you can use this tool to calm your system down and deal with the real issues at hand. Eventually, you will be able to employ this exercise immediately after a difficult moment, or maybe even while it's happening.

After another week or so, take a look at your drawing. How does it appear to you now? You may discover that your body landscape has changed a bit. Your self-image may be clearer. The problem areas may be more informed. Feel free to take your pencil or color pencils and add to or reconfigure your drawing.

Danger

Monique's parents were very caring. So caring that they never let anything ever happen to her. Her mother carried her all the time, even when she was old enough to walk. Anytime Monique started to cry, a parent came running over to find out what was wrong. When she finally learned how to walk, her parents hovered. If she walked too close to the sharp corner of a table, her mother would leap from her chair, exclaim, "Watch out, Monique! You could hurt yourself!," and yank the startled child to safety. When Monique wanted to ride a bike, her mother tearfully refused. "You could fall down and crack your head open. Some car could run you over!" Forget girls' softball. "You could get hit by the ball!" By the time Monique went to college, she knew that the world was a dangerous, unpredictable place. And even though she loved literature, she majored in business, because it was safe.

I began to work with Monique when she was almost fifty years old. She drove only when she had to, and well below the speed limit. Each time she got out of the car, her jaw was so tight from tension that she had a headache. She walked with a stiff gait, staring at her feet so as not to trip over anything and fall. Whenever she got to the end of the room, she needed to touch the wall or an object to assure herself that she had made it. She gripped the chair back as she went to sit, so as not to lose the chair on the way down. Monique was in constant pain.

As we worked together, Monique became aware of her walk, her posture, her shallow breath. She noticed her fear of falling in every step. Very slowly, she began to relearn how to use her pelvis, how to move her shoulders. Sometimes she walked almost normally after a session, but to her it felt like staggering, and she would quickly tense up again. Eventually, she learned to enjoy this staggering, and even laugh with delight as she swung her hips, discovering in the process a whole new aspect to femininity.

Why is it that some people choose skydiving and other people are frozen on the couch? We looked earlier at how childhood experiences mold our perceptions of the world. Monique's parents startled her so many times that she was stuck in a variation of the Startle Reflex posture.

A child's nervous system develops according to the kind of stimulus it receives at certain key growth periods. A protein sheath called myelin coats the nerves. It helps conduct the messages in the sensory/motor system. Children have bursts of myelin growth from birth to adolescence. There is a folk saying that by the time a child is twelve, he is "crystallized"—that is, his habits have been formed and nothing can change them. By constantly having the same idea, the fear of injury, reinforced, Monique's entire nervous system came to revolve around that possibility.

The good news is that habits *can* be changed. Scientists

have discovered that the act of learning helps create new neural pathways. It's kind of like upgrading to a new operating system on your computer. Research has confirmed that learning also grows new brain cells. In a recent issue of *Science* magazine, Princeton scientists Elizabeth Gould and Charles Gross reported "that the formation of new neurons or nerve cells—neurogenesis—takes place in several regions of the cerebral cortex that are crucial for cognitive and perceptual functions. The cerebral cortex is the most complex region of the brain and is responsible for highest-level decision making and for recognizing and learning about the world."

If you feel that your life is filled with limitations due to fear of injury, you may want to try some of the following exercises.

→ *Connecting With Your Breath*

There's a lot of talk these days about the value of breathing—as if we don't do it! If you weren't breathing, you wouldn't be here. However, it is often difficult to allow full and functional breathing. Remember that part of the Startle Reflex involves holding the breath. Anytime something delicate or dangerous is required, the body tends to hold its breath—doing fine jewelry work, peering through a microscope, aiming a camera or even a gun. But when the nervous system interprets logging online as a reason to hold its breath, or chopping onions, or lifting a cup to the lips, then you start to suffer from oxygen deficiency. Carbon dioxide builds up in the lungs, creating lactic acid in the muscles. You feel stiff and sore. Your movements become labored. How much more difficult it is to skip from stone to stone across a pond, or negotiate a narrow hiking path, or even maneuver through rush hour traffic, if the body feels uncooperative and achy.

Find a comfortable position—laying down is best, but you can do this exercise sitting in a chair. Just take a few moments and notice your breathing. Don't try to change it or improve it. Just notice how you breathe. How long is each inhale? Is it longer or shorter than the exhale? Do you hold your breath after the inhale, after the exhale, or after both? Which one do you hold longer? The natural breathing pattern is inhale, hold, exhale, hold. Each person has a different rhythm. Just take a moment to notice yours.

Now see if you can sense where there is movement as you breathe. Do you feel movement in your abdomen? Feel free to put your hand on your abdomen to check. Many people have been told that the "proper" way to breathe is abdominal breathing. That's fine, but other areas of the body are involved as well. Don't try to make movement happen, however, just notice it in yourself.

Notice if there is movement in the chest. Do you

feel anything happening with your ribs? What about your back? Do you feel your breath moving your shoulders in any way?

Now intentionally stop the movement of your abdomen. Even if you feel there was no movement there, at this time hold your abdomen tight and don't let any movement happen there. In fact, place your hand upon your abdomen. Many people think they're inhibiting movement but they're not; they just aren't used to sensing themselves. So make sure your hand is not rising or falling. You can breathe everywhere else. For some people, this will feel difficult, if this is your primary area of moving while breathing. See if you can find movement somewhere else. Try it about five times. Then breathe normally. Try the same thing with your chest. Place your hand on your chest to check if you have actually stopped movement. You may not think you use that part; perhaps you think of yourself as a "belly breather." But you'd be surprised that there is some movement. Once again, hold your chest in place for about five breaths, then return to normal breathing. Try the same thing with your shoulders. And your back. Each time, intentionally inhibit a part, then let it go.

Sit quietly for a moment. Then notice: Has your breathing pattern changed at all?

When you find yourself about to deal with an uncomfortable situation—walking down stairs, driving in the rain, going to an unfamiliar place—pause and spend a few minutes doing the above exercise, or part of it. You will see that making this investment makes the action a little easier and a little less painful each time you do it.

Taking full, even breaths also affects the nervous system. It responds to changes in your breathing, interpreting what it thinks is happening. If the breath is short and rapid, your nervous system can only think that you are in danger. Easy, full breaths signal the relaxation response—all's clear. You stop firing adrenaline and the other neurotransmitters that excite the fight-or-flight response and regain balance.

Control Issues

Sometimes fear of injury keeps you from trying things, from going for a walk to extreme skiing. Now, of course, there's no reason to court danger, and for most of us avoiding extreme skiing is probably a wise choice! But some people won't go in the water for fear of drowning, won't go for a hike for fear of falling off a cliff, etc. Most of these fears come from a need to control.

No one wants life to be out of control. But with maturity comes the knowledge that you can't control everything. If you try, it will only make you very tense. Whether your need to control comes from a chaotic childhood, memory of an accident, or just your personality type, when it begins to limit your choices you close down the possibilities of a fully functional life. Moshe Feldenkrais used to say that in any situation, you should be able to see at least three choices. If you think about going into the city, and the only choice you see for unfolding events is that you're going to get mugged, you have allowed your fear to control you while fooling yourself that you have control over your destiny. How can you reintroduce choice, how can you let go of the illusion of control?

As with any fear, you can be living in complete denial of your fear of losing control. You may have cleverly arranged your life so you never have to go to the city. Or you may never go swimming, saying you just hate the water. Not only have you limited your options in the world, you don't even know you're doing it. If this is the case, you may want to go back to the exercises in chapter 2, "The First Step," page 23). Once you can see that you are afraid, you can begin to work on creating choice.

One year, I was traveling through India. On a whim, I joined a trek through the southern Indian mountains. After several hours, we came to a river. It was a lovely river. But there was no bridge. There were a few slippery rocks. The group stopped dead. The guide, who was wearing plastic sandals, just walked through the river. Several of the young women hopped from stone to stone, holding on to the guide, laughing as they slipped and got wet. Now, I've gone on hikes before where I've fallen in the water and had to walk for several hours in wet shoes. I also know I can be clumsy at the most inopportune times. I considered my options: I could walk across the stones without incident. I could walk across the stones and fall in. Or I could take off my shoes and just walk across the river. Which I did.

One young woman stood frozen on the bank. She did not want to take off her shoes. She did not want to fall in. She had only one choice that was acceptable to her, and the odds were not good. Gritting her teeth, she grabbed the guide and began gingerly moving from one rock to another. She gripped him in such a way that it was difficult for him to keep his balance. One particular stone required a bit of a jump. She stood there a long time, on the verge of tears. When she finally jumped, her foot slipped. She was so frightened, she fell on the guide, knocked him over, and landed on a rock, spraining her wrist. Her pack weighed her down, so that she flailed like a beached whale in the water. When we finally got her, soaking wet, to the bank, she was battered and bleeding and covered with leeches. She had lived out her worst-case scenario.

If she had been willing to accept other choices, she might have avoided injury, or even losing her balance. But her fear of injury was so intense, she put herself in jeopardy. When old people feel unstable, they become so rigid that they are more prone to falling and injury. By learning to create choice—physically through improving physical balance, mentally through creating options in each situation, and emotionally by recognizing that nervousness or anxiety is only one choice—

the possibility for injury is reduced. You don't have to leap into the deep part of the water if you are afraid to swim. There are other choices.

→ Discovering Your Options ⟩

We'll start by exploring choice simply, through movement, and then see how this can apply to your fears. Lie on your back with your legs stretched out. Take a moment to check in with how your body feels in contact with the ground. Now bend one leg and stand your foot (*see* illustration 4.1) on the floor. Which foot did you choose? Do you always start with the same foot? What would it be like to use the other foot instead? Play for a moment, bringing one foot to a standing position, then let it come back down to the floor, then bring the other foot to a standing position and notice if they feel different. Can you choose either foot?

Now, keep one foot in the standing position. Begin to gently lift the hip of your standing foot off the floor (*see* illustration 4.2). Several times, just lift the hip and let it come down. Can you notice how you do it? Or does it just do itself? Do you push with your foot? Is your thigh involved? Do you rotate your pelvis? Squeeze your buttock? Tense your back? What does your abdomen do? You don't have to have answers, and you don't have to move all these parts. These are just some of the many actions that take place when you move your hip.

Let's look at some other options. No matter how you

have been lifting the hip, try lifting it only by pressing your foot to the floor. First of all, is it possible? Easy? Difficult? Are you able to not squeeze your buttock? How high do you need to lift your hip to know that you are moving it? Does this affect the direction of your hip movement? Rest a moment. Now try the same thing by adding your upper leg (*see* illustration 4.3). How do you add it: Do you tense your muscle? Do you lengthen the femur downward to the knee? Is this familiar, or weird? Let your leg slide down and rest.

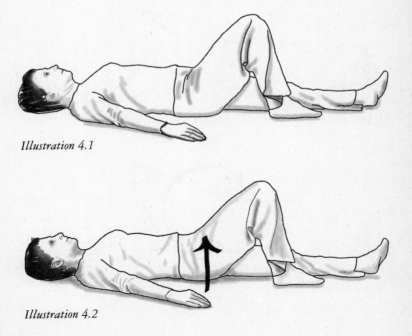

Illustration 4.1

Illustration 4.2

Bring the same foot to a standing position again. Now raise your hip by squeezing your buttock. Tighten it as much as possible and lift it several times. Is this familiar? Easy? Difficult? Let it go. Now lift the hip by rotating/twisting your pelvis to the other side (*see* illustration 4.4). It's as if one side of the pelvis gets lighter, and the other side gets heavier. Nothing else. Can you do this without tensing your buttock? Now rest.

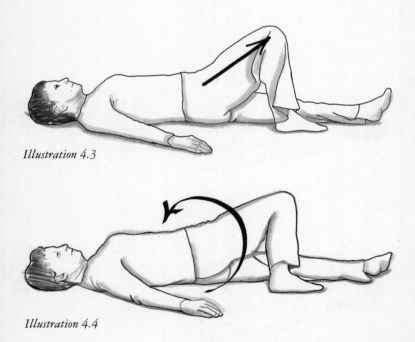

Illustration 4.3

Illustration 4.4

For many people, the easiest choice for moving the hip is tensing the buttock. Tensing the buttock is a very effective way to get instant action, but it's hard work! If you tense your buttock while laying on the floor, odds are you tense your buttock all the time in order to get where you want to go. Or, when you repeat this exercise, you may notice that you tense your neck, your jaw, or some other part of your body. This tensing is your body's attempt to control your movement, just like your trying to control your environment. It's not only not useful, it can be harmful down the line. Physically, always controlling from the same part leads to postural problems and wears out the related joints. Always trying to control your life by limiting choices makes you less open to change and growth, putting you at risk in the event of any kind of shock. By exploring other choices for movement, you can make your movement easier. Paradoxically, when you see how limiting choices is about the illusion of control, you actually develop greater freedom and safety!

Once more bend the same knee and try lifting your hip without thinking. Has the movement changed? After resting, feel free to try this on the other side.

→ Life Choices

Now take your notebook or a sheet of paper and write down something you won't do out of fear of injury. Not something unrealistic like daredevil cycling but something from your ordinary life. For example, I won't drive during rush hour because I'm afraid I'll get hit by a car. Now let's look at choices. According to your scenario, you have only two options: stay home, or endanger yourself in traffic. How could you create a third choice? Don't feel like you have to come up with the definitive answer or even a logical one. Your list might look something like this:

1. Repeat safety affirmations as I drive.
2. Drive only side streets.
3. Pull over every time I get really nervous.
4. Go to driving school.
5. Hire a driver.
Etc.

They may appear to be silly choices. That's okay. They may appear impractical, like trying to lift your hip with just your foot. But by exploring choices, you will discover solutions. Instead of being frozen, you will begin to take steps toward living a more courageous life. And, perhaps, it will suddenly become as easy as lifting your hip.

Checking In

You may want to take another look at the drawing of your body that you started back on page 50 and see what it says to you now. You may even want to draw a whole new image.

Perhaps your shape has changed. Or the dynamics. Remember, it doesn't have to be anatomically correct. You can have different shapes, different colors, even flying arrows. In one workshop, a woman began with a body drawing that was just a big square, and by the end of the day she had become a shooting star.

5. *Fear of Failure/Success*

Falling/Failing

There is a Greek myth about a young boy named Icarus whose father, Daedalus, made wings of wax for himself and his son so they could escape from imprisonment in the labyrinth of Minos on the isle of Crete. Daedalus admonished Icarus not to fly too close to the sun because the sun would melt the wings. But Icarus didn't listen. He flew higher and higher. And the sun's heat, sure enough, melted the wax wings and down he tumbled to his death in the sea.

When I was growing up, this myth was used to teach children that you should obey your parents. And parents, of course, are the first people to teach us how to fear. Remember Monique back in chapter 4? It was the parents' anxiety as Monique was wobbling on her first steps that sent her shoulders up to her ears. Not to mention how bad she felt as she crashed to the ground. Monique grew up with a fear of falling, of taking the wrong step.

I look at the myth of Icarus now and see that it's about how parents set limitations with double messages. I mean, really, why would a parent give a child wings and then tell him not to aim too high? We want to soar! But someone is always there to say, "Uh-uh, you better not. You'll fall!"

Sometimes I feel that my life is a series of trapeze swings. I'm either hanging on to a trapeze bar swinging along, or, for a few moments in my life, I'm hurtling across space in between trapeze bars. . . . And so, transformation of fear may have nothing to do with making fear go away, but rather with giving ourselves permission to "hang-out" in the transition between trapeze bars. . . . It can be terrifying. It can also be enlightening, in the true sense of the word. Hurtling through the void, we may just learn how to fly. —*The Essene Book of Days*

Of course, it's not always the parents. Sometimes we do it to ourselves. I once had an interesting conversation with a thirteen-year-old girl, Bethany. Her parents, divorced, are both highly regarded performers who have made many sacrifices in order to fulfill their creative dreams. They are not financially successful, however.

I asked Bethany what she was going to be when she grew up.

"A corporate lawyer. Preferably with an established firm."

"Oh! You like the law?"

"Corporate lawyers make a lot of money."

"But, why do you want to be a lawyer? Does it excite you?"

"I dunno."

Now, Bethany has a lot of artistic ability and seems to really glow whenever she's involved in a show. So the whole thrust of our conversation really surprised me.

"Well, to be a corporate lawyer, you're going to have to do contracts, mergers, paperwork, work long hours to climb the corporate ladder. I mean, you seem to really like theater and writing. Why a corporate lawyer?"

Bethany turned to me and gave me a patient look, like I was a somewhat daft five-year-old. "Look, I've seen what comes of pursuing your dream. Look at my parents. No thank you. I'm going to have a sensible life."

Bethany won't wear wings even if her parents beg her to!

A colleague of mine once said he thought Icarus's problem was that he didn't know how to fall properly. One of Moshe Feldenkrais's definitions of maturity is to not be afraid of failing. Is it a coincidence that these two words— *fall* and *fail*—are only different by one letter?

'Tis better to have loved and lost / Than never to have loved at all.
                                                    —TENNYSON

Falling Metaphors

We use the word *falling* in dozens of ways in our daily language. Yet we rarely connect it with the physical sensation that takes place when you actually yield to gravity and crash-land. Just for fun, go back to some of the fears and/or dislikes you addressed on page 37. Now see if you can find a sentence that connects *falling* with any of them. It may not work for every one, but it gives a different perspective. For example: I don't like paying the bills because I feel like I'm *falling* into debt. I'm afraid to confront Jerry because I can't handle a *falling-out*. I don't like parties because I'm afraid of *falling* on my face.

Dynamic Stability

Two powerful forces are at work in the universe: one is movement, the other stability. Each has its advantages and disadvantages. In times of extreme dynamism in a society, we see unrest, revolution, even chaos. For some people this is an exciting time. Old attitudes and rules fall by the wayside. Witness the French Revolution, the Bolshevik movement, or even something small, let's say a change in how the Board of Ed in your town addresses the issue of classroom size. When the revolution has achieved its desired results, we enter a period of stability. The problem with stability is that it leads to entropy. The longer something remains the same, the more it decays, becomes rigid, sometimes even turning into its opposite—the idealism of Bolshevism turned into the Stalinist terror. In order to maintain the status quo, society or the individual imposes an order to "keep things as they are." Meanwhile, things fall apart underneath, leading to collapse.

Many times, fear of failure/success is related to fear of change. Moving from static to dynamic can be dangerous. What if all hell breaks loose? What if change makes things worse? What if the chaos causes madness? Better to keep things—lousy as they may be—as is.

According to many ancient myths, there was a time when trees could freely move about. There are even Celtic epic poems of wars among various kinds of trees. The recent film version of Tolkein's *Lord of the Rings* trilogy has revived this myth of the walking trees. All of these myths eventually end with trees deciding to stay put for various reasons. For stability, they have exchanged their dynamism for rigidity. They are at the mercy of the ax, and the weather, falling instead of moving on. If it can happen to trees, it can happen to you.

No one wants to lose an investment. By deciding to move on, you may lose everything you've come to rely on. If you stay in place, you can't fail. Or succeed.

Swaying

One of the easiest ways to fall is to try to stay in one place. The human body was designed for movement and our systems were designed to keep moving ahead. A perfect example of this is the periodic phenomenon of the Buckingham Palace guard keeling over. Even standing still is never *really* still. Measurements using force plates have demonstrated that we sway in a figure-eight pattern. According to Dr. Reuven Ofir, a physical therapist and Feldenkrais teacher, "The sway is caused by a continuous synergistic flow of contraction/relaxation of the leg, ankle and feet musculature, which by timed contractions, assisted by the array of valves in the veins, helps pump blood back up to the heart and head. If insufficient blood (oxygen and glucose) reaches the brain, the sway increases until the center of gravity of that poor guard tilts beyond the boundary of his base of support."

→ Catching Yourself

Stand still and close your eyes. After a moment or two, notice whether you feel any movement. How does it feel to sway? Is it fun? Disturbing? Do you feel vertigo? Open your eyes and intentionally sway forward and back, side to side. How far do you go before you feel you need to catch yourself? How do you catch yourself? You need to take a step. Walking is actually falling. Each time you take a step, you are falling and catching up. Do you catch yourself stiffly? Does your knee bend? Can it? What does your torso do? Is it scary? Fun? Now look at your attitude toward moving ahead. Is there a correlation between your feelings in this exercise and your feelings about the things you fear?

Satyajit Ray, a renowned filmmaker, made *Aparajito,* about India in the 1920s. It shows the struggle between a mother, locked in her old ways, and her son, determined to go to college and evolve. Without him in her life, she wastes away. Neighbors come with invitations. People offer help. She refuses them all. She prefers to sit and wait for her son's return, because all she wants to do is serve him. She is unable to move on, afraid of innovation. She finally dies alone, having refused to change.

→ *Moving On*

1. Write down six things that you'd like to change in your life. Maybe you're sick of a certain behavior, or maybe you've been procrastinating instead of taking care of business. They can be seemingly minor things: I want to start untying my shoes at night instead of just kicking them off. Now write alongside each entry on your list the payoff for just staying in place.

2. You don't want to create chaos. You want a state of dynamic stability, a safe place where you can move toward change without losing your footing. So pick one of the items on the list and change it. Again, it can be the smallest thing: I will close my dresser drawers. By changing one thing, you begin to change the whole structure.

3. Go for a walk. How do you react to this instruction? Do you hate walking? Do you walk

quickly, trying to get it over with? Do you dawdle? Do you go the same route every time? How you approach walking is how you approach your life. As you walk, experiment. Change one thing about your walk. Maybe the way you swing your arms. Maybe the way your heel strikes the ground. Maybe the route you take. Notice what takes place inside you when you change one thing.

Dynamic stability allows you to be more flexible. It's a lot easier to jump out of the path of a moving object if you are not rooted in the ground. Remember, everything changes, whether you want it to or not. It's up to you whether that change is growth or decay.

There is a saying that we learn more from failure than from success. The truth is, even though failure is often painful, it gives you an opportunity to clarify your goals, refine your approach, become wiser, though not necessarily sadder.

Jeffrey came to see me with multiple problems: chronic pain, fibromyalgia, Crohn's disease. For fifteen years he had been struggling with varying degrees of debilitating pain. Although he had been a top executive for a major corporation, he no longer worked. In fact, he'd been out on disability for over nine years. In that nine years, his pain had become his career. He spent all day of every day running to various therapists (except psychotherapists, who he considered a waste of time), doing exercises and sitting with ice on various parts of his body. He walked like a stick man that was animated by a windup key. Everything moved jerkily around a rigid torso. One day, as we worked together, he asked me what I thought differentiated a successful person from a failure.

"What do you think?" I asked, curious about where he was going.

"Well, I've done a lot of questioning about this. I mean, in my job, I saw lots of very talented people who seemed to never get ahead. And after really studying them, and talking to others, it seems that successful people have a kind of confidence, a willingness to take a risk, to perhaps fail, look foolish. Those who stay below their level are those who were afraid to come forward with the dangerous idea, the wild proposal, to invest in that new concept. They were comfortable."

I totally agreed with Jeffrey. Then my task became to make Jeffrey aware that he had become comfortable in his "pain career" and was afraid to take the risk, to try to live his life without fearing that he would be punished by another onslaught of pain. And, of course, that meant that he would have to risk reentering society, something I knew he was absolutely terrified to do.

After we had significantly reduced his pain, we began changing small things. He had always insisted on keeping his shoes on until the moment he lay down, for fear of pain. Slowly, I encouraged him to take a few steps in socks. He was surprised that it was okay. This made him willing to try other things. He began to make one call a week to old colleagues. Then he had lunch with them once a month. Each small change caused a difference in his attitude, his bearing, and, eventually, his life.

We all know people who are comfortable in their misery. The friend who won't exercise even though he's at risk for a heart attack and wheezes at every step because he's so overweight. The coworker who is a brilliant writer but sits all day doing data entry because she's too afraid that her writing will be rejected. The cousin that drives a jalopy held together with duct tape and coat hangers because he's "got sentimental attachment, and, besides, I know all its quirks, and who would buy it?" . . . the list goes on. It's a kind of hiding, this miserable comfort. Mice, if left in a box long enough, refuse to come out. Prisoners don't want to leave their cells for the sunshine of freedom. Old people don't want to leave their rockers.

A friend of mine went to visit her deteriorating grandmother. She found her sitting in her armchair, staring at the TV. "Come on, Grandma! I'll take you to town!" she exclaimed brightly.

Grandma looked up at her as if she thought her mad. "Why should I want to go to town? I was there once!" she retorted.

In the previous chapter, we talked about the need for choice in a fully functional life. Another by-product of limiting yourself is that your world becomes incredibly small. It can start with a sore left shoulder. You don't lift with that shoulder. Then you stop using your left arm for carrying the groceries. Pretty soon, the left side becomes so stiff, it's hard to walk. So you walk less. Then you stop going out. If you don't use it, you lose it. It is easy to become accustomed to unacceptable conditions. And, of course, as life becomes more unbearable, you begin to lack the strength to change. If you put a frog in hot water, it jumps out. But if you put him in cold water in a pot on the stove, then turn on the heat, he'll sit there and boil to death.

If you don't put yourself out there, you can't fail. If you don't write the book, quit the job, move away—if everything stays the same—you never have to suffer bad reviews, unemployment, loneliness. That's what your nervous system would have you believe. But the truth is, it won't get better. Just like the frog, you'll cook in your misery, your options will evaporate as you get more and more entrenched in your protective habits.

➔ Jumping Out of the Pot

Have you grown accustomed to your misery? How have you limited your options? Write down six things that are stopping you from moving on. They could be physical, emotional, professional. Your list might read:

1. My migraine headaches
2. I need medical insurance

3. My mother needs me
4. No one will read my book anyway
Etc.

Realize that all of these could be strategies you are employing unconsciously to protect yourself from failure.

Review the exercise for creating options in chapter 4, page 66. Now look at your list above to see if you can list three options for action next to each complaint. For example:

3. My mother needs me
    1. Get someone to help her out for a few hours a day
    2. Speak to family members and enlist their support
    3. Talk to Mom and explain that you need your free time

Your choices may seem unrealistic at first. But just write them down at this time and look at them at least once a day.

S-U-C-C-E-S-S

When King Midas got his wish that everything he touched be turned to gold, he was ecstatic. He had achieved his life's dream. But we all know that his very wish turned against him, turning everything, even his food, into gold.

What happens when you get the girl of your dreams, reach the pinnacle of your career, win the highest honor? The saying "The higher you go, the harder you fall" rings deep in our psyche. Going back to Icarus, if he had never flown he would have never crashed.

Throughout his childhood, Stefan heard the same phrase, "You are so useless, you'll never amount to anything!" His father was a bitter man who had never realized any of his dreams, and he was unconsciously passing his legacy on to him. Stefan is an extremely talented artist with a variety of skills. However, each time his career seemed about to take off he sabotaged things. Or it seemed as if his best efforts were rewarded with setback. How *could* he succeed? He'd prove his father a liar. That would tumble the entire house of cards Stefan's life was built upon. The last thing Stefan needed was to incur his father's rage, even though he was already dead. Stefan's fear of success was disguised by his hard work and "bad luck." No one would ever accuse *him* of being afraid.

Stefan began to explore movement lessons when nothing seemed to help his aching lower back. Often, during the rests, he would find himself in imagined conversations with his dead father. Or an image of himself as a child swam up. Often he realized he was holding his breath, or tensing in that very spot in his back. Gradually, Stefan was able to let go of the pain in his back. At the same time, he moved from being angry at his father to realizing that his father hadn't been intentionally malicious. He had just been repeating a pattern that had probably gone on for generations. Stefan forgave his father. He forgave himself. He sees now how he literally got in his own way, and he has begun the adventure toward success.

With success comes responsibility, the attention and expectations of others. It's a lot easier to sit in your room and muse about what might have been if you had only made that call, gone to that audition, tried to manufacture that product. At least you don't have the world banging at your door putting all kinds of expectations and pressures on you. No one expects much from a failure. When you're a success, people suddenly become your best friends because they want to bask in your success. Not only that, but when you're successful everyone is watching, waiting for you to blow it. How can you know who your real friends are?

Katie was a beautiful girl, slim, a champion skier, an accomplished gymnast. Her father had raised her to be perfect. So perfect that when she spent her first weekend away with a boyfriend, she never let him see her go in the bathroom for fear he would think she was coarse, merely human. Men were always hitting on her, even after she was married. She tried to be all things to all people—attractive, active, vivacious, fun. Then she was in a motorcycle accident and hurt her back. "You'll be on your feet in no time!" "We expect you on the slopes any day now!" "Boy, will your family be grateful when you're able to take care of them again." Katie stopped walking. Her legs froze. She blamed the accident. She blamed the medical diagnosis, which was never clear—a vague statement about MS-like symptoms. She spent her time watching *Oprah* and QVC, eating massive amounts of ice cream and growing bigger every day.

We began working together on the tension in her shoulders. Because her legs were untrustworthy, Katie tensed her shoulders and neck each time any movement was required. Soon we discovered that she could move her pelvis and waist, something she had forgotten once she became wheelchair-bound. Different movements reminded Katie of dance moves, ballet postures, skiing techniques from her youth. Many of the somatic memories led to recollections of her demanding father, her critical mother, the first husband who nearly beat her to death because her makeup wasn't perfect for a dinner party . . . After much work, she admitted being terrified by the thought of having to go back to being the perfect wife, the perfect mother, the perfect athlete, the perfect beauty. By recognizing her fear of the demands of success, she felt freer. She stopped smoking. She went on a diet. She began to do volunteer work. She began reclaiming her life.

Symptoms of Fear of Success

Take the following test. If more than half of the answers are true, you may want to look at the possibility that fear of success is stopping your progress.

1. You start lots of projects and never finish them.
2. You get embarrassed when anyone compliments you, perhaps even contradicting him.
3. If someone says something nice about your work, you immediately make a mistake.
4. You get bored with jobs or relationships quickly and quit, or get someone angry so that you have to leave.
5. When you see famous or successful people in public, you think, "God, I could *never* do that."
6. When things start going well, you say things like, "Yeah, well, any day now the shit's gonna hit the fan."
7. It seems like every time success beckons, something goes wrong, or you get the carpet pulled out from under you.
8. Every time you seem to get ahead financially, an unexpected disaster occurs—the car explodes, you get sick, the ceiling falls in—so that you're broke again.
9. You overcommit to too many things, so that nothing can be done well.
10. Deep down inside, you know you don't deserve success. (Come on, be honest.)

Evelyn grew up in semipoverty. They bought day-old bread and went shopping at thrift stores before it was trendy. She vividly remembers her parents' anxiety as they struggled each month to pay the bills, answer the creditors' phone calls, and eat potatoes for dinner night after night. She made a resolution to become rich when she grew up so that she would never experience this type of anxiety again.

Evelyn pursued a career in advertising, growing wealthy and secure to a point where she no longer felt the wolf at the door. And then the work stopped. The phone went dead. As they say in show business, she "couldn't even get arrested." The anxiety level escalated as her hard-won savings disappeared, her gym membership lapsed, her massages canceled. The good life had evaporated.

Just at the edge of desperation, Evelyn got a call for a job to be account executive for a major ad agency. It was actually a huge leap up the career ladder. It was for a very prestigious client, yet a product she was completely unfamiliar with marketing, but she had been out of work for months so she flew to Orlando for the interview, where she learned the salary would be four times what she had been making before.

As she drove in her rental car back to the airport, she was overwhelmed with anxiety. Was she competent enough? Likable enough? And then she heard a little voice inside of her. "You'll never amount to anything," said this voice from the past. "You're just a no-good bum, you don't deserve anything." She clenched her fists on the steering wheel so tightly her knuckles turned white, and she began to shout, "I deserve to be rich! I deserve to be successful! I deserve to be rich!" She rolled down the windows and shouted at the top of her lungs through the Florida streets.

Evelyn is now an advertising VP, one of the few women who has made it through the ranks in the business.

The following movement exercise can help you study your attitudes toward failure and success.

✦ Non-striving ☽

Lie on your back. Take a moment or two to sense the weight of your body on the floor. Notice what parts of your body are comfortable. Are there any parts that don't quite touch the floor? That seem tense? Just notice.

Bend your knees and bring your feet to a standing position on the floor, about hip width apart. Interlace your fingers and put them behind your head. Fold your elbows in around your face and gently lift and then lower your head several times, as if you wanted to see your knees. (*See* illustration 5.1.) As you raise and lower, notice: Are you able to do this without straining? How high do you need to lift your head in order to know that you are lifting?

Rest a moment.

Now bring your knees up over your chest. Interlace your fingers behind your head again. This time, lift your head and move your elbows toward your knees. (*See* illustration 5.2.) Repeat several times. Allow your movement to be soft. Notice your breath. Do you inhale or exhale as you do the movement?

Rest.

As you're resting, just reflect. Were you striving to touch your knees with your elbows? Did touching your

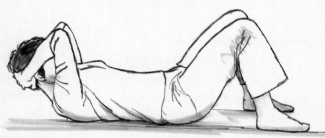

Illustration 5.1

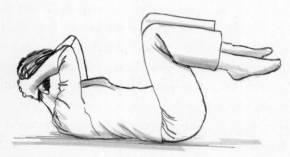

Illustration 5.2

knees become a "goal"? Did you succeed? Did you get frustrated trying to do it? Are you tired now? If you did touch your elbows to your knees, are you satisfied? Irritated? Was it a struggle?

Bend your knees and bring your feet to a standing position again. This time, bend only your right knee over your chest. Hold on to your knee with your right hand. Put your left hand behind your head. Gently move your left elbow toward your right knee. As you do this movement, ask yourself: When do I consider this movement a success? Is it in the doing? In the touching? Am I trying to do it well? Or am I doing it for myself?

Rest. Notice your thoughts.

For the next few minutes, play around a little with this movement. You can switch arms, bringing your right elbow to your right knee. You can do the same sequence going to the left knee. Throughout the process, give yourself time to question: Are there moments when I feel like I'm failing to do this correctly? Where do I feel that? Am I trying to prove something? To whom?

After exploring this movement for about two or three minutes, let it go, stretch out your legs, and rest. Don't think, just drift.

Now bring your knees up over your chest. From between your legs, place your right hand behind the fold of your left knee. Cross your left arm over your right arm and place your left hand behind the fold of your right knee. Holding on to your legs, stretch one leg downward toward the floor, and then the other. As you do this movement, your arms alternately lengthen. Let this movement evolve into a rolling movement from side to side.

Rest.

How did you do? Were you angry that the instructions weren't clear? That there was no illustration? Were you anxious about doing it correctly? Was it fun? Satisfying?

Once more, interlace your fingers behind your head. Bend your knees over your chest. Bring your elbows and knees together. What is it like now? How do you feel about it?

Who would think that one could experience anxiety, anger, satisfaction just by bringing the elbows and knees together? Yet these small movement explorations can help inform you about your attitudes toward failure and success. The way you respond to movements in this environment is the way you respond to life's challenges. In the laboratory of self-study, you can safely come in touch with attitudes and emotions that stand in the way of your success. If you felt nothing at all during the above exercise, be patient. Try it again at a later time. Many times, emotions are buried so deeply it appears that nothing is going on. Emotions are always present. Your brain is constantly pumping out hor-

mones and other chemicals that keep an emotional life going. If you feel nothing, you are just not yet hearing the conversations taking place inside you. You are not a failure.
Don't be afraid to try again.

Success is never final and failure is never fatal. It's courage that counts. —JULES ELLINGER

6. Phobias

Claustrophobia, arachnophobia, agoraphobia, vertigo—the list goes on and on. These are the dramatic fears, literally. Horror movies tap the deepest part of our nervous system, stimulating our most primal fears. A person who has become paralyzed by a phobia lives in a nuclear reactor. All someone else has to do is push the button and the chain reaction begins. He cannot stop it, only helplessly watch, or get totally sucked into the absolute terror of the particular phobia.

You get into a crowded elevator and you can feel the discomfort of others crowding around you, invading your space, the doors closing, the awkward silence. But the chemical factory of your body/mind system continues normal production—you know in a second the bell will ring, the doors will open, you will step out into the lobby. For someone with a phobia, the factory has decided that the elevator, or the supermarket, or the mountaintop, is life-threatening. Beyond life-threatening, because in a life-threatening situation you would be roused to defend yourself, to escape. However, in a claustrophobic situation, there is no escape. The combination of helplessness and fear is what brings on a panic attack.

This is an oversimplification, and there are many books available that explore these issues in more scientific detail. Working with a good psychotherapist can often help you discover the origin of your phobia and develop behavior-modification approaches to control it. The question is, how can you use the intelligence of your body/mind system to bring more safety into your world?

More commonly, the side effect of phobias is that you avoid places and situations that can trigger your reaction. You won't get on an elevator. You won't go to the supermarket. You don't go for a hike. This naturally limits the choices you have in life. It's not uncommon for a small fear to grow to a point that nothing feels safe outside your house. You end up avoiding everything. You end up shutting yourself out of life's pleasures as well as life's pains.

Again, each phobia comes from a very healthy fear response to danger. If we jumped off cliffs, we would die. And it's true, people *can* die when trapped in an elevator. But with a claustrophobic reaction, your response mechanism has gone haywire. Pain studies have revealed that different people experience different levels and types of pain for the same injuries or diseases. One theory is that it's not the actual tissue damage that causes the pain, but how the nervous system responds and signals the organism.

The relatively new field of psychoneuroimmunology is beginning the exploration of this relationship between the mind/body and well-being or illness. If you break the term *psychoneuroimmunology* into its component parts, it literally means how the mind connects with the immune system. In the early 1980s, several groundbreaking research scientists discovered neuropeptides and neuroreceptors in other parts of the body. Neuropeptides, according to Dr. Candace Pert, a maverick scientist who discovered endorphin receptors in cells, are "those chemicals secreted by the brain and known to mediate mood and behavior. . . ." She discovered that these very chemicals were "clearly signaling . . . cancer cells via their receptors and causing them to grow and travel, or metastasize, to different parts of the body." She, along with others, tracked the relation of the endocrine system, which comprises all of our ductless glands and their secretions, with the brain and the immune system.

The discovery of neurotransmitters and receptors has affected all aspects of health research. Neuropeptides in the stomach have given a new meaning to "having a gut feeling." The Institute of HeartMath states that neural pathways between heart and brain affect our behavior and our health.* Fear, as was discussed earlier, is the firing of complex neuro-

---

*Rollin McCraty, Ph.D., "Influence of cardiac afferent input on heart-brain synchronization and cognitive performance," Institute of HeartMath, Boulder Creek, Calif. Presented at 11th World Congress of Psychophysiology, Montreal. Published in the *International Journal of Psychophysiology* 45, nos. 1–2 (2002): 71–73 (www.heartmath.org).

transmitters and hormones in order to assist survival under dangerous circumstances. The signals sent along these neural pathways are much quicker than your intellectual mind. And for good reason. If you had to think about what to do as you swerved to avoid a drunken driver, you'd never make it.

A couple of other aspects of phobias need to be understood before you can enter into a constructive healing process. First is the self-fulfilling prophecy. For everyone, there is a first time for a panic attack. You're driving down the highway and, suddenly, for no reason, you become terrified. Your heart begins to pound, sweat beads on your lip, your hands start shaking. You pull over, sit there and tremble. And then it's over. Physiologically, a panic attack can only last around twenty minutes. At that point, the body stops producing adrenaline. It always passes. But even if you know that, your body can't accept such a rational thought.

So the next time you have to drive, you begin thinking about what happened last time. You are nervous even before you leave the house. As you approach the spot on the highway where it happened, your knuckles are white from gripping the steering wheel with nervous anticipation. You hold your breath. And guess what? You have another attack. Once the pattern of panic begins to take hold, your body makes it part of the program.

The "factory" now turns this pattern into a physiological habit. This transformation is the second important factor that needs to be understood. Even if you try to tell yourself "I will not freak out, I will not have a panic attack when I drive," the body responds to everyday triggers—putting on your coat, picking up your keys. It begins manufacturing the adrenaline necessary to reproduce what it has interpreted as part of the experience of driving. The nuclear meltdown begins. Panic becomes a habit, and driving becomes a phobia. When a phobia becomes habitual, it's only a matter of time before you stop driving altogether . . . or getting into elevators, or even going into buildings that have elevators. Eventually, you may not want to go out at all. Free choice has once again been eliminated.

Now, it is true that some panic disorders are the result of a chemical imbalance. While it's possible that it is a chicken-and-egg situation—that is, panic causes hormonal problems or hormonal problems cause panic—you should see a doctor to rule this possibility out.

> He who is afraid of a thing gives it power over him.
>
> —Moorish proverb

Breaking Phobic Habits

If you suddenly find yourself in a situation that triggers your phobia—say, you're going for what was supposed to be a little hike through the woods and suddenly you find yourself on a high precipice—it's difficult to remain calm. The combination of shock and the unsafe environment is too much for the system. So then is not the time to try to change your phobia response.

As mentioned before, once the fear button is pushed it's virtually impossible to stop the reaction. So the way to begin to free yourself is to practice where it's safe. You don't start learning to play basketball by leaping out onto the court with the New York Knicks. Your first violin lesson will not go well if it's onstage at Carnegie Hall. You practice in the relative safety of a studio, with a teacher or coach you trust. You take the time to train your body to be able to respond, so that when you're on the court and the ball is passed to you your nervous system can make the appropriate choices.

Learning how to create other options in a moment of panic is the same as learning how to execute a quick pass to the right guy while thousands are watching and screaming at Madison Square Garden and millions on TV sets around the world. You must practice, practice, practice in order to triumphantly score the point. And if you don't score the point you don't freak out, you just go on with the game.

Even if you practice approaches to working with your phobia, there will be easy days and difficult days. Under stress, your nervous system can default to an older pattern. But your ability to recover will have improved. If you are seeing a counselor or taking medication, do not stop treatment without his or her approval. As I said before, phobias and panic attacks are often the result of complex chemical imbalances. The following exercises are intended to assist you in your recovery and not as a substitute for treatment.

Return to the Breath

Many of the previous exercises can be very helpful in addressing your phobias. For example, the breathing exercise in the last chapter can help you understand what happens to your breath in a moment of terror. By learning how to breathe properly while relaxed, you can use your breath to calm yourself when faced with one of your phobias.

Change Your Focus

If you put your mind on something else, you can sometimes calm yourself down. Here is a movement that helps you turn your attention toward yourself in a way that "fools" the nervous system into reducing anxiety.

→ *The Bell Hand*

Find a comfortable position, either sitting or laying down, where you can close your eyes and feel safe. Very gently, bring the thumb and other fingertips of your right hand together until they touch. Your thumb and fingers should not be pressing or straining in any way; it's as if they are all coming together to greet each other. Then gently let them open apart. (*See* illustration 6.1.) Repeat this movement, bringing the thumb and fingers together to touch, then gently opening them, until you've established a softly pulsing rhythm.

Continuing the hand movement, turn your attention to your breath. Have you been able to breathe freely while doing the movement with your hand? Is the rhythm of the movement the same as the rhythm of your breathing? Can your breath and your movement be independent of each other without strain?

Play for a few moments, seeing if you can keep your hand movement and your breath soft and free. Each time you notice your hand getting tense and your breath becoming compromised, or you find you are locked in identical rhythms for breath and hand, pause, return to just breathing, and try again.

For the first session, trying the above synchronization should be enough. If you feel you are comfortable with this movement combination, you can begin to experiment with adding more complexity to the exercise. Once you have the hand pulsing easily, and your breath is regular, try slowly turning your head from side to side. If that synchronization becomes easy, then see what it's like to slowly stand up and start to walk around the room while continuing the pulse.

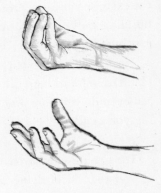

The Bell Hand exercise is a simple neurological way to calm the nervous system. Wilder Penfield, a neuroscientist, first mapped the brain

Illustration 6.1

and its relation to motor function and sensory reaction. In his map of the motor and sensory cortex, located in the parietal part of the brain, the area relating to the thumb and fingers is huge. They are important receptors of information. Each time your thumb and fingers all softly touch each other, you are sending a series of signals to the brain—an A-OK. You can't do this kind of movement while running for your life: terror does not allow you to pulse your hand; however, pulsing your hand can keep terror at bay. As you become more comfortable with using the Bell Hand at home, in your safe environment, you can begin to take it with you when necessary.

First of all, if you are nervous about an impending situation—say, you are starting to panic about having to drive to the supermarket—take five minutes before you start to get ready and do the Bell Hand exercise. You can continue with it all the way to the car, always listening to your breath, keeping everything soft, not rushing. Don't attempt to do the exercise while driving, but should you start to feel panic building pull over and pulse until you feel calm enough to continue.

No matter what your situation, you can apply the Bell Hand exercise to help calm down your nervous system. You can even do it before going to sleep at night if fear is keeping you awake.

Try a thing you haven't done three times. Once, to get over the fear of doing it. Twice, to learn how to do it. And a third time to figure out if you like it or not.

—VIRGIL THOMSON

Exploring Mindfulness

There is a term in meditation called *mindfulness*. The ultimate intention is to know yourself. Most people think of meditation as something you do sitting on a cushion, with bells, soft music, dim lights. While this practice is very useful, there is another way to use mindfulness to understand habits. The Dalai Lama said in his book *An Open Heart*, "You can meditate while driving or walking, while on a bus or on a train, and even while taking a shower."

It doesn't matter whether the habit is cigarette smoking or fear of heights, the same approach applies, albeit in reverse. We spoke in the last chapter about how changing one small thing changes everything. Therefore, when working with physical habits, you must *allow* the habit to change. One tool that helps is mindfulness. Forcing yourself to change one habit can create other, less attractive habits to take its place. For example, many people who force themselves to quit smoking start eating. People who force themselves to go on a diet can develop a habit of irritability. And so on. So if you're going to work on changing the habit of panicking, you have to be careful not to force the change.

One way to do this is to create a pause in the habitual response. For example, a person always has a cigarette immediately after eating. If he could decide in advance on a specific amount of time—say, thirty seconds, two minutes, whatever, during which he would delay his cigarette—and during that time try to observe what he is thinking, feeling, and sensing, he may discover that the urge to smoke has changed. It may have diminished. Or he may notice how tense he is, and that smoking makes him feel like he "fits in." Or he may notice his breath and then sense how it changes as he inhales. The important thing in this exercise is not to try to *stop* the habit but merely to *observe* it for a few minutes. Moshe Feldenkrais often said, "If you know what you are doing, you can do what you want." If you are not clear about what is taking place in a moment of panic, there is no way to free yourself from it.

Interestingly, the very act of observing your habit creates a change. There is a law in physics called the uncertainty principle, developed by Werner Heisenberg in the late 1920s. It's really about the nature of particles and waves, their motion and trajectory. It was discovered that you can never predict whether you're going to observe a particle or a wave, because they change according to who's watching. Scientists disagree on whether this phenomenon has anything to do with our ordinary lives. But if you start to observe your habits, you may discover there's something to it. My friend Jerry once summed it up like this: "The nature of the phenomenon changes based on the attitude of the observer."

So how does all this apply to your phobia? Like a scientist, you can begin to observe the phenomena surrounding your fear. It's not just an intellectual observation, however. Remember, the particles and waves change based on who is watching, so the attitude of the observer is paramount. Your attitude comes from your emotions, your mind, and your body. As you notice these parts of yourself, something is bound to change.

✦ Increasing the Safety Zone

This exercise requires something besides observation: intention. You have to decide in advance how you are going to approach your fearful situation. Let's go back to the elevator. Where does the fear begin? In the parking lot? The lobby? When you hear the elevator bell ring? If possible, pick a time when it's not really essential to use the elevator: a day off, lunch hour, after work. As you drive into the parking lot, or walk toward the building, notice yourself. What is your breath like? Are your palms sweating? What are you thinking? If this is too much to attend to, then stop. Literally. Just stop and stand there for a moment.

When I was a young performer, I once blanked out on stage during a solo piece, and forgot what to do next. It was only for a second, but it felt like an eternity, hundreds of people's eyes upon me. Afterward I went up to the director of the company and asked him if that ever happened to him, and, if so, what did he do. He laughed. "Of course it happens! What do I do? I stand there and think. 'What was it I was supposed to do next?' The audience assumes it is the character that is thinking and completely accepts the pause!"

You may think that passersby are staring and judging, but the fact is that everyone occasionally stops and thinks: Do I have my keys? Was that store I wanted to go to on 59th Street or on 57th? Did I call Mary? Right, right, I did. So you are standing there, noticing. It looks the same! Now slowly approach the thing you fear—the top of the stairs, the door of the building. *Don't think about what's going to happen when you get there because you're not even going to try to get there today. It's not about forcing yourself to get there.* Notice when you get to the point where the panic builds. Now step back. That's all. Just step back to where it feels safe. And notice. How does your breath change? Again, what are you thinking?

Never try to push past your comfort level. Don't even take it to the edge of your safety zone. The space before the edge is where learning takes place. Moshe Feldenkrais stressed that as soon as you go to your limit, possibility for going further has been destroyed. As long there is further to go, you can change your definition of a limit. So just back off when it feels like enough. And now let it go. Don't repeat it. Don't think about it. Go on with your day.

When you feel ready, try the whole thing again. Notice: Do you stop at exactly the same place each time? Can you feel any interest or curiosity in the next step, or does it remain a closed door? At some point, you may find that you can begin to approach your fear. You may begin to hear thoughts that are creating your fear. The point is not to *trigger* the panic, just observe the conditions that invite it.

Each time you try the preceding exercise, you will learn something more about your habit of panic. Thoughts will come up: about your past, trying to explain your feelings, and about the future, trying to rationalize your feelings. Just observe them and you'll see that these thoughts are helping to create your fear. You will notice sensations—sweaty palms, tensed shoulders, shallow breath. Don't try to make them go away. Just stand there and observe them. Like naughty children, they will get embarrassed and disappear. And if you never make it into the elevator, that's okay. I don't plan on going bungee jumping anytime soon, either. The important thing is not that you "succeed" at what society expects you to do. The important thing is knowing yourself, your perceived limitations and the choices available to you at any given moment. If, some day, driving becomes more important than your fear of driving, you will choose to turn the key. You may even discover that, indeed, the emperor has no clothes. The terrible wizard is just a little old man behind a curtain. Your fearful monster is just a shadow projected on your psyche.

"Why, you're no wizard at all!"

—DOROTHY, *The Wizard of Oz*

7. Fear of Abandonment

To be an outcast, to be rejected by your tribe, to be thrown to the wolves: these are primal fears that speak directly to our fear of death. In aboriginal tribes, one of the most terrifying punishments is to be cast out into the wilderness, to be exiled. Without the protection of the tribe, you're as good as dead.

Now, of course, we are modern people, right? There are no monsters in the woods waiting to devour us. If we are rejected by parents, lovers, friends, coworkers, we can just go somewhere else. And yet, so many people don't. Fear of abandonment is at the core of destructive friendships, abusive relationships, boring marriages, even meaningless jobs. Fear of rejection keeps people from trying something new, from following their hearts, from making a change.

Krishnamurti stated that when one goes against the tribe, one risks being alone. Loneliness for many people is death. And yet the root of the word alone is *all* + *one,* originally meaning that to be by oneself was to be complete. Being without others is lonely, yet to be truly complete you must be alone! So how can we resolve this paradox?

Even our society exemplifies the paradox. America often is considered the land that rewards the rugged individual. The pioneer, the venture capitalist, the guy who went against the tide of opinion and made his fortune, or revolted against oppression, or freed the slaves. At the same time, women for centuries were not given equal rights and *had* to marry in order to survive. Workers were promised medical benefits and retirement security *if* they toed the line, caused no friction, stayed faithful to their employers. Most people fear that individuality, outspokenness, or vision get rewarded with a pink slip. Truth is, people who try to go their own way rarely find support in the beginning. When a person succeeds, becomes a millionaire, even famous, in spite of cultural limitations, then everyone jumps on the admiration bandwagon. So most people play it safe—stay in the dead-end marriage, stick with the family business, keep the hateful job. It's safe, and you remain part of the tribe. Or is it so safe? Society has changed radically since these family and business values first surfaced. Nowadays, neither marriage nor a job is any guarantee of security. There is no safety in toeing the line and doing what is expected. So what are you afraid of?

In his book *Quantum Healing,* Deepak Chopra uses the terms *self-referrent* and *other-referrent.* When you are other-referrent, your value is based on how others perceive you. If you are self-referrent, your value comes from within yourself. As long as you are other-referrent, you need to please your father, your boss, your wife before you please yourself. You can't make decisions for your best interests because you might get thrown out of the family, fired, divorced. By becoming self-referrent you run the risk of feeling abandoned and rejected.

Loss of Love

In some ways, you could call fear of abandonment the core behind fear of success and fear of failure. When we go back to the essential principles of love and fear, we can see that fear of abandonment is not simply about survival but about loss of love. Ask any comedian. She will tell you that the absolute worst feeling in the world is when people start walking out on your act. The audience doesn't love you anymore. In fact, when the act is dying, many performers experience the symptoms of a panic attack: racing heart, prodigious sweating, shortness of breath, inability to think clearly. There's even a name for the sweat: *flop sweat.*

For many people, the connection between love and abandonment starts at an early age. Most people grew up in a home that unwittingly promoted conditional love. Even if your parents were the most loving people you could imagine, their approval or disapproval affected your child psyche deeply. After all, if they were unhappy with you they might not love you anymore. And if they didn't love you anymore, they might throw you out. Or leave you.

Remember this? "Come on, now! If you're not over here by the time I count to five, we're leaving without you! You'll have to figure out how to get home all by yourself, that is, if we let you in the house. One, two, three, four, five. Okay. That's it. Good-bye."

Children develop many survival tactics to make sure they're safe. One is to try to be as much like Mommy and Daddy as possible. After all, if I walk like Daddy, and think like Daddy, how could he not love me?

As an adult, you no longer fear abandonment by Mom and Dad, but your behavior has become programmed, and not just by fear but by everything you picked up from them.

I was walking through Manhattan one day and passed a exclusive little boutique on Madison Avenue that features expensive knickknacks. In the window was a needlepoint pillow embroidered: *Mirror, mirror on the wall, you are your mother after all!*

So how do you find the real you?

Fear of Lack/Self-Esteem

So many times when I ask people "What are you afraid of?" I get answers like "He won't think I'm pretty enough," "They'll hate my manuscript," "I'm going to look like an idiot," "I'll run out of money." These fears all issue from your self-esteem, or lack of it.

There is something that drives every human being: a constant wish to improve, to enhance. More is better. Keep up with the Joneses. He who dies with the most toys wins. This need for more is hardwired into our nervous systems, and at its best has resulted in spectacular civilizations and marvelous technology, and at its worst cheating, murder, war.

Things are magnified even more by advertising, by the media—designer clothes, muscle cars, celebrity worship. Even toothpaste is glamorous. You can never be smart enough, rich enough, thin enough . . . good enough. This feeling of lacking something often turns itself into fears that stop development of you as a person.

This is an insidious form of fear of abandonment. Self-esteem is a currency, like money itself. If you have money, brains, looks, talent, you can get what you want. If you lack it, you feel left out in the cold. You lose your power. Health activist Helen Caldecott has drawn a parallel between the rise in incidence of prostate cancer in men and the loss of money or job. As men lose their self-esteem based on diminishing financial or professional success, she suggests, this loss of potency often seems to result in medical problems. For women, beauty and brains are symbols of power. A beautiful woman holds men in her thrall, and if she's smart as well she can conquer anything. Loss of these powers can also lead to health issues. Money, beauty, brains are the myths we are taught as children. The key to overcoming fear of not having or losing any of these powers is to learn to use what you do have and not worry about what others say you don't have.

Interesting, isn't it, that in biblical times there was a coin called the *talent*!

In the book of Matthew, there is a parable of a man who is going away. He gathers three servants and gives them each a talent. While two of the servants invest and double their money, the third servant is afraid: he fears losing his money; he fears his master's wrath should he lose the money. He takes his talent, therefore, and buries it in the ground until the master returns. The master rewards the two servants who took a risk and invested their money. The one who buried the talent he kicks out of his house.

The obvious interpretation of this parable is that you should invest your money. But you also can look at it in another way: each person is given a talent in life, and the choices are either to develop that talent and profit from it or to bury it.

A dear colleague and student, Mary Marcus, told me the above parable. She is a Presbyterian minister who always longed to be in the theater. She told herself, however, that the ministry is a safe way to satisfy her wish to communicate, to be "on stage" each week in front of her parishioners. Mary also admits that she hates the Matthew parable because, deep down inside, she feels that by making the choice she did she has "buried" several of her talents.

Mary began taking Feldenkrais classes in order to relieve some of the tension she always felt in her shoulders and neck. As the neck became freer, Mary's walk began to change. She felt less stiff as she approached the pulpit. She stopped relying on her meticulously written notes and began to look people in the eyes as she delivered her sermon. And then one day, to illustrate a point, she burst into song. As she left the pulpit, a colleague remarked how gracefully she walked. Mary had found a way to use her talents as currency in her chosen vocation.

There are many wonderful books available to help you to make more money, be smarter, enhance your beauty. But far more useful than trying to acquire what you feel you lack is to recognize what you have. And often the fear of lacking obscures the wealth of having.

There is a Japanese folktale about a man who had a huge, hideous growth on his face. Fearful of ridicule and rejection, he avoided everyone in the village and spent a miserable, impoverished life as a maker of charcoal. Each day, he'd go into the woods and gather sticks, bringing them home, and burning them into charcoal, from which he and his wife eked a meager living.

One day, while gathering his sticks, a terrible thunderstorm appeared out of nowhere. The man dashed for shelter inside the hollow of a large old tree. When the storm finally passed, it was night. Just as he was about to venture out into the night, he heard some very strange sounds. Right in front of his eyes was a bizarre gathering of hobgoblins, dwarves, and other mutated creatures. Some had three legs; others had eyes dangling from their heads on stems. These creatures were various colors, some were furry, all were unquestionably hideous from the ordinary human point of view. It was a party, and soon drumming and dancing ensued. The charcoal burner watched in delight as the music built and the hobgoblins danced. His feet started to itch to join them. But he was afraid they might devour him. He stood in the tree hollow, listening to the music, until he couldn't bear it anymore. He burst out of the tree hollow and began to dance. He was brilliant. The hobgoblins all stared in admiration as the charcoal burner flipped and twirled, basically stealing the show. When the dance was over, the creatures begged him to return the following evening, they had never seen such a talented human. They demanded a pledge for his return. To them, his unsightly tumor was an incredible asset. They insisted he leave it behind to ensure his return! Suddenly, his growth was gone. He ran home, the happiest man in the world. But even better, the bottom of his charcoal basket was filled with gold. The charcoal burner became the wealthiest man in the village. By letting go of his fear of rejection, he had discovered his true currency: his talent for dancing. And he learned that even his tumor had value—for the right audience.

When paralyzed by fear, be grateful for what you *do* have. Fearing rejection because of a perceived inadequacy causes both physical and emotional insecurity. How can you possibly go into that meeting if you think everyone will look only at the zit on your face? How can you stand up straight in front of them if you think they will laugh at you? Experiencing gratitude is like being in a state of grace. You become centered, sure of yourself, because what you have *is* enough.

The following exercise can help bring you back to that centered state.

→ *Prayer Hands* ⸜

Almost every culture has a gesture of putting the two palms together in front of the chest. In India, it is used as a greeting while saying "Namaste" [pronounced Na-ma-stay], which loosely translated means "I salute the divine in you." Western religious traditions include a variation in their prayer rituals. As was mentioned earlier, placing the fingers together sends a powerful message to the sensory cortex. François Delsarte, a celebrated teacher of oratory in the early nineteenth century, stressed the power of gesture in communication. He codified every part of the body according to what he called "The Principle of Trinity": the head (mental), the trunk (emotional), and the limbs (physical), which were then further subdivided into specific details of gesture. According to this gestural science, hands to the heart is a way to connect the mental and the emotional sides of the self. He felt the hands were an expression of the thoughts, and the chest the seat of the emotions.

Sit comfortably in a chair and slowly bring your

palms and fingers together in front of your chest. Allow them to barely touch, then separate them slowly a few times. Feel how sensitive they have become. Now bring them together so that everything is in solid contact. Begin raising your hands, still palm to palm, toward the ceiling and back down in front of your chest. Notice your breath. Where do your eyes go? Your head? Repeat this several times, taking in whatever information comes up.

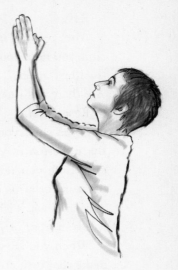

Illustration 7.1

Rest.

Once again bring your palms together. This time as you raise your hands and arms, raise your head and eyes. (*See* illustration 7.1.) As your hands return, bring your head and eyes to neutral. Does this feel any different? Is this what you were doing before? What do you feel in your face? In your belly?

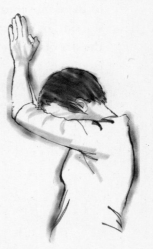

Illustration 7.2

Rest.

After resting, try the same thing, but this time each time you raise your hands up lower your head and eyes (*see* illustration 7.2). Feel what happens to your back. Are there any images that come up for you?

Rest again.

If you wish, you can repeat this exercise, alternating the direction of your head. Allow yourself to exhale each time you raise your arms. Feel how this movement of the arms is connected to your back and chest. Any time you wish, take a moment to pause with your hands in front of your chest.

When you are about to go into a meeting, need to make that call, are afraid you will be inadequate, take a moment and place your hands together and do a few of these movements, sensing your breath. You can go full out, or you can do very tiny movements—it's not the size of the movement that counts but the attention paid to it.

As the movement centers you, perhaps gratitude will replace the feeling of lack that inhibits your possibility.

Fear of the Unknown

> And the day came when the risk it took to remain tight inside the bud was more painful than the risk it took to blossom.
> —ANAÏS NIN

One of the scariest parts of abandonment is being tossed into the unknown. Going back to the tribal outcast, or the exiled prisoner—they were forced to travel, alone, into often dangerous and unpredictable territory. They had no friends, often no belongings, and no way to predict the future. Every day presented new risks and challenges.

In the same way, we often stay in situations and relationships that are no longer healthy simply because they are known. It may be miserable, we tell ourselves, but at least I know this misery. People who hate their jobs are often devastated when they get fired because even though the job was hell it was predictable. When you are thrust into the unknown, the illusion of control is gone.

While you are responsible for your actions and your beliefs, you have no control over the weather, accidents, disasters. This was grimly borne out on September 11, 2001. Those who died, those who overslept and didn't make it to work that morning, or got caught in a traffic jam on the way in, none of them had gotten up that morning and said "I know what's going to happen today." They could say "I won't go to work today" or "Think I'll sleep in." But the consequences of their actions could not be predicted.

There are philosophies that say you do choose your own

destiny, that people "unconsciously" choose life or death each day. The key word is *unconscious.* As you become more aware of yourself, you may indeed notice how you choose situations that affect what we call "fate," and how your fears determine your choices.

There is a tale of a Sicilian girl named Catherine. She lived in a sumptuous palace with her wealthy father. One day she was visited by Fate, who asked her if she wanted her good fate at the beginning of her life or the end. After a pause, Catherine decided that she wanted a good fate in old age. Immediately things started going wrong: her father lost his fortune, thieves ransacked the palace, her father died and she was left penniless in the street. She found employment as a servant, but as soon as she started to feel comfortable Fate came in and tore the place apart, each time forcing Catherine to flee in terror. It wasn't until Catherine summoned up the courage to confront Fate that things changed. Even then, Fate worked mysteriously. For instance, Catherine was handed a skein of silk thread, and when the King announced that he needed a shirt woven of a particular color it was up to Catherine to weave the cloth . . . You know how the story ends. Fate was just waiting for Catherine to change her own destiny.

Embracing Change

When someone stays in a dysfunctional relationship only because there is a sense of security in knowing how each day will turn out, the result is usually disastrous. The thing you feared the most often comes to pass: you get dumped; you're fired; you get sick and then are abandoned. You're unwillingly thrust into the unknown.

The ultimate dysfunctional family is found in the Old Testament. There was a family of brothers whose youngest was named Joseph. Because Joseph was the youngest, and also the most talented, his father adored him and his brothers hated him. Joseph also had a gift: he could interpret dreams. Unfortunately, most of his dream interpretations went completely unappreciated by his jealous brothers, but Joseph was so adored and protected by his father that his life was as secure and cushy as it could be and it didn't matter. Then one day the brothers grabbed him and threw him in a hole, leaving him to die, but then changed their minds and sold him to a bunch of camel traders. One misadventure led to another until Joseph ended up in prison in Egypt. It was in Egypt, because of his skill interpreting dreams, that he eventually became Pharaoh's right-hand man.

Your gift, your talent, may be totally unappreciated where you are right now. The question is, do you wait until you get dumped, fired, abandoned, or do you make the leap?

Leap, and the net will appear.   —GOETHE

Baby Steps to Freedom

Learning to love yourself, to trust your inner instincts, to rely on your talents, is lifelong work. Learning to embrace the unknown has been the journey of seekers throughout history. The effort requires the greatest courage of all, and will continually challenge you at different levels for the rest of your life. *What Are You Afraid Of?* can only begin to direct your search. At the very least, you will learn to recognize this most insidious fear. At the most, you will have some tools to aid you in your adventure.

Changing Your Attitude

Carol loathed her husband's cousin Antonio. He was boorish and shallow. Every year, there was a huge family party at Antonio's house. Carol never wanted to go, complaining the whole time about what a lousy time she was going to have, how unendurable her husband's relatives are, etc. Sure enough, every time she went to the party everything was exactly as she expected.

We don't need to analyze Carol's issues about Antonio. If we simply operate from the premise that every emotion stems from love or fear, we certainly can agree that Carol's reactions did not come from love. What we can explore is the possibility of allowing the unknown into Carol's life. If Carol could set aside her fear of having a bad time at Antonio's, she might discover the opposite, or, at the very least, learn something about herself.

→ Exploring Attitude

In the morning, choose an arbitrary time during the day, say, 2:05 P.M., when you're about to go on break or maybe take a walk. Then set the alarm, if you need to, to remember. It's easier if you choose a time when you know you'll be alone. At 2:05, stop and look inside yourself. What is your attitude about the next hour? Is it horribly predictable? Are you a nervous wreck because you know your boss didn't like your presentation and he's going to cream you? Are you looking forward to that quiet cup of tea as you check your e-mail? Just notice if somewhere inside yourself you've created some kind of anticipation and belief about the next hour, that something in you "knows." Then go on with your day. Over the course of the week, notice how many times things go as you imagined and how many times they don't. If you can, try to remember how you felt, without judgment, just trying to see if there are any connections between your attitude about what you "know" and what really happens.

→ Sensing the Unknown ⟩

The challenge of this exercise is not to read ahead. Try to experience each thing as it happens. Lay on your back. Review in your mind the Discovering Your Options exercise you did in chapter 4, page 66. (*See* illustration 7.3.) Slowly draw your right leg up so that your foot is in a standing position, then begin to raise and lower your right hip. Take a few moments to remember the feeling. Change the standing leg and try it with your left hip. See if you can just "experience" yourself without any agenda. Make sure you rest after doing the movement a few times. If you've straightened your legs, bend your left leg again and put the foot in the standing position. Keeping your right arm flush to the floor, extend it diagonally above your head. (*See* illustration 7.4.) Now, begin a reaching motion with your right arm, as if you are laying on the beach and you lazily are

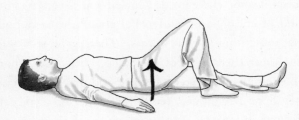

Illustration 7.3

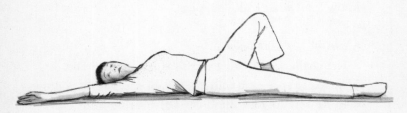

Illustration 7.4

reaching for some suntan lotion up there—you know it's there, somewhere, but you're too lazy to look. Reach and release several times. Notice where your thoughts are going. Do you want to know what happens next? Are you impatient and wanting to get to the end already? Or are you able to just experience this moment?

So now it appears that the suntan lotion is eluding your grasp, so turn your head and look up toward the reaching hand. Each time you reach, turn your head, look up. Each time you release, return your head to the center. Can you feel how including your head when looking toward your goal affects the center of your torso? Notice how just using your eyes to look to the goal changed the entire quality of your reach. And you're not even reaching for a real bottle!

Rest a moment.

Now, resume the same position: left knee bent, right arm extended. As you reach, turn and look, adding the movement you did earlier of raising the left hip off the floor. How does that affect your reach? (*See* illustration 7.5.)

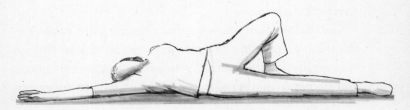

Illustration 7.5

Keep going. Keep pushing with the hip. Where does it take you? Do you end up in a different orientation? Are you still on your back?

You may still be on your back pushing with your hip. Or you may be on your side. Or you may have rolled over on your stomach.

Let go of these movements and rest. While resting, notice how you are feeling. Notice any emotions that may have arisen—from reaching, from pushing, from trying to figure out what was next, where to go next.

Often, when I teach this lesson, there is a yelp of delighted surprise as someone unexpectedly lands on his stomach. Almost immediately, other members of the class see what happened and figure out how to roll over. But they are already moving to the known—they saw a result and decided to duplicate it. It's a valid experience. It's nice to feel the shift from back to stomach. But why weren't they able to just roll in the first place? *Because they were stuck in their expectations, in the known.* When you have an idea of what is supposed to happen, there is no room for surprise. There is no chance of hurting yourself, but there is also no chance for unexpected pleasure.

Embracing the unknown is risky business but rarely life-threatening. You are merely risking the loss of your illusion of control. You are opening yourself up to new experience. You are not living in the future or the past—you are experiencing *now*.

So do not be concerned with the fruit of your action—just give attention to the action itself. The fruit will come of its own accord. . . . When the compulsive striving away from the Now ceases, the joy of Being flows into everything you do. —ECKHART TOLLE

8. *Unavowed Dreams*

arlier, we talked about payoffs—why some people pursue their dream of skydiving, why others stay in their dead-end jobs. Many people wake up at age forty or fifty with the devastating realization that, somewhere, they abandoned their cherished dream. Whether it was to be an architect, a fireman, a dancer—somehow it appears that life circumstances interfered. Because of thwarted dreams, people walk around harboring hidden wounds that prevent a joyful life. Remember the wounded king in the story of Parsifal: He never spoke of his wound even though it was there for all to see.

Of course, not all dreams get buried by fear. Parental pressure, accidents, a death in the family, an unexpected pregnancy are just a few life circumstances that alter the course of your life. Fear, however, often does play an important part in deferring dreams, and often in unexpected ways. Remember the story of Stefan in chapter 5? He couldn't be successful because it would prove his father a liar. The image of your parents can make you afraid to pursue your dream. And even if the course of your life was deflected not by fear but by circumstance originally, you may experience fear, even disease, as a result of suppressing that dream.

Rita is a dedicated and talented R.N. with a real gift for healing. Her childhood was filled with physical and sexual abuse. She turned this experience with abuse into a deeply compassionate wish to become a holistic nurse working with energy medicine. While enrolled in the holistic nursing school of her dreams, she entered an abusive marriage and had a child. Things got so bad, she left her husband and was forced to quit school in order to work and raise her child as a single parent. As the years went by, one thing after another got in the way—her child needed college tuition, she had a new husband, they had a home to pay for, now she has to babysit her grandson . . . A few years ago, Rita started to get sick; pain and anxiety ruled her days. She wouldn't go out in the evening for fear of having an accident, or getting sick the next day. She was afraid to lift her grandson because it hurt too much. She was afraid to tell her husband she needed more time with him because she was afraid he would turn abusive like her last husband. She felt tyrannized by her boss at work, who kept threatening to fire her for being sick. When I asked her why she didn't just go back to get her holistic degree, she just sighed. "I just can't. It's too late. There's no time."

Rita's posture was the posture of defeat. Her eyes were always downcast, her head tilted a little to the side, her shoulders were slumped yet rigid. She was constantly protecting her solar plexus, literally keeping her hands or a pillow in front of it; she didn't feel safe unless covered. Her breathing was shallow and erratic. All of these conditions fed on each other. As mentioned earlier, shallow breathing causes lactic acid buildup in the muscle tissue, resulting in pain. Also, rounded shoulders compress the organs and limit breathing, thereby depressing the immune system.

By developing awareness of her body, and gently restoring a sense of ease, Rita has begun to emerge out of this dark time in her life. As her posture improves, she is feeling more assured, more willing to look others, and life, in the eye. With improved breathing, the pain is subsiding, giving her more freedom to try new things. She is taking time off and exploring the possibility of going for that certification in holistic nursing. She has asked her daughter to hire a sitter, and her husband is taking her on some of his business trips. She's not out of the woods yet, but at least she's found the path.

Whether fear is the cause or the result of a dream deferred, until fear is recognized you will carry it around with you, even protecting it the way Rita protected her solar plexus, unable to move ahead. It's not about forcing yourself to go take dance lessons at age fifty because you wanted to be a ballerina at age five. It's about acknowledging the dream and discovering what you can do about it today, without the interference of fear.

> It is not true that people stop pursuing dreams because they grow old, they grow old because they stop pursuing dreams.
> —GABRIEL GARCÍA MÁRQUEZ

Remembering Your Dream

Many times, a dream has been so deeply buried that you don't even remember it. Remember Monique? She wanted to study German literature, but her fear of poverty made her study business instead. She had stored her books from college in boxes and forgot all about them. But recently, she started to reread them. Her conversation is no longer just about market trends and investments; we're having dynamic discussions about Kafka and Goethe. She's considering going into teaching economics instead of continuing in the corporate world. Her teaching will be informed by great writers, not just dry statistics.

Recovering your dreams can be scary. What if you suddenly admit that you never really wanted to be a dentist but a sculptor and here you are twenty years later with an upper-middle-class lifestyle, three children headed for college, and you're president of the Rotary? Do you throw it all away, or is there some elegant way to integrate the earlier dream with the current reality? Instead of fearing that you are in an all-

or-nothing situation, spending time with your body/mind in personal exploration can help you choose a path that is courageous *and* satisfying.

The following two exercises are designed to work with the nonverbal parts of yourself—how the buried dream resides in your posture, movement, and tensions. These movement sequences, and others like them, often help to open the door first to questions and then to insights regarding the suppression and perhaps ultimate realization of dreams.

→ *Feeling Your Power/Freeing Your Spine* ☽

Eastern medicine stresses that a rigid spine is a sign of poor health. Certainly, a tight spine is prone to injury. An inflexible spine undoubtedly creates limitations in changing direction, let alone the ability to move ahead (or anywhere, for that matter!). It compromises one's sense of safety: with limited range of motion, how can you respond effectively to life's stresses? The movement of the pelvis is intricately connected to the spine's flexibility. A frozen spine often results in a frozen pelvis. A frozen pelvis can indicate impotence, an inability to act, a lack of freedom. When deferring dreams, the spine and/or pelvis can become inflexible, literally holding you back. Give yourself permission to fully explore the sensations that come up during the following exercise—without analysis. *If nothing comes up the first time, try doing the entire sequence again in a few days.*

Lay on your back. As you have in previous explorations, take a few minutes to observe how you are at this given moment. Notice your breath; notice how you are contacting the floor. Bend your knees and put your feet in a standing position on the floor about shoulders' width apart. Begin raising your pelvis, and then your back, up off the floor, then lower them down again. (*See* illustration 8.1.) You don't have to spend time with your back in the air; it's simply the *action* of raising and lowering the pelvis and back you're interested in. Notice how it feels. Is it smooth and comfortable? How far up can you go easily? When do you inhale, when do you exhale? Do you ever hold your breath? Notice how your spine lifts. Does it come up all at once? In sections? One vertebra at a time? Or some combination? Notice if you feel any tightness in your back or shoulders. Can you do anything to make the movement easier?

Now stretch your legs out and rest.

Stretch your arms out to the sides, aligned with

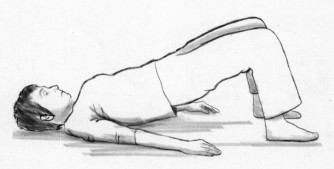

Illustration 8.1

your shoulders, with palms up (*see* illustration 8.2). Bend your right leg and place your right foot in a standing position on the floor. Begin tilting your right leg over toward your left leg. Repeat several times. When your leg has tilted as far as is comfortably possible, leaving the right foot on the floor, can you somehow stretch your leg to lift the right hip off the floor? (*See* illustration 8.3.) Think about some of the strate-

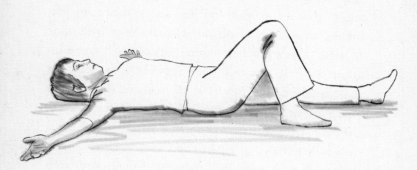

Illustration 8.2

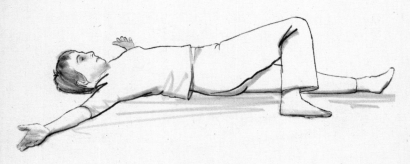

Illustration 8.3

gies you discovered for lifting the hip in earlier exercises. Try pressing your foot a bit into the floor. Lengthen your thigh and your knee. How could you easily lift that right hip?

As you are doing this movement, notice: Are you trying really hard? Can you lighten up? Can you exhale as you stretch? Are you tightening your buttock? Do you need to? Do you feel anything in your back? Your ribs? Your neck? Your head? Does the movement feel pleasant or does it feel stressful?

Rest quietly with your legs stretched out. Let your mind drift for a few moments. Perhaps your attention will be drawn to the bodily sensation. Or you may tune in to some background thoughts that are swimming up to consciousness.

When you feel ready, try the above sequence with your left leg bent, tilting your leg to the right. Take as much time as you need to rest afterward, again allowing your thoughts to roam freely, following them with your attention.

Bend both knees and bring both feet to a standing position about shoulders' width apart. Tilt both knees to the right. If it's comfortable, roll your head to the left as your knees go to the right. (See illustration 8.4.) Now see if you can lift your left leg off your right leg. Let your legs open really wide apart as your left leg travels to the left, pulling the right leg over. (See illustration 8.5.) Don't move both legs together; instead, allow a space in between your legs as they pass from one side to the other. What does it feel like to let your legs be so far apart? Is it even possible, or are you putting on the brakes with your inner thighs? Does it feel safe? Liberating? Terrifying? Is there a way to make this exercise fun? Babies learn to move by playing. Can you let go of judgment and seriousness and turn this movement into play? Roll from side to side any way that feels good.

Rest for a few moments with your legs long.

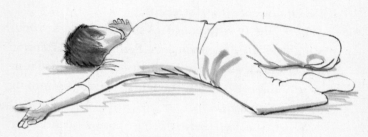

Illustration 8.4

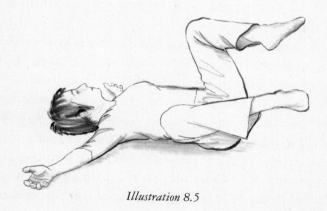

Illustration 8.5

Once again place your feet in a standing position about shoulders' width apart. Go back to your original lifting the pelvis and back movement. Notice how it feels now. Has anything changed or is it exactly the same? Is it possible to sense a difference, or is it hard to remember what it was like? What is your emotional state at this moment?

Now roll to your side and stand up. Walk around a little. Is your walk different?

You can remain standing, or sit down. Picture yourself as you were when you were eight years old doing something you loved. What was it? Now, take paper or notebook and just write—don't edit.

If you have time, go outside for a walk. Allow your mind to wander even as you sense the movement of your pelvis and spine.

You can repeat this exercise as often as necessary. You may find that each time you visualize yourself in the past, each time you sense yourself in the present, you are experiencing something different. Eventually, like a puzzle, all the pieces fall into place.

Playing for a Living

We have become so accustomed to having to work to earn money so that we can enjoy ourselves that we have forgotten the simple joy of doing something just because it's a pleasure to do so. We all have vague childhood memories of "playing." But what kind of play was the most satisfying?

Ivan spent his childhood combing through garbage cans, coming home with walkie-talkie entrails, cathode tubes from discarded hi-fis, miles of telephone wire. He would sit in his room and create mechanical robots. Once he wired the house with speakers and when his parents started arguing he bellowed into a microphone, "This is God talking. You two better stop fighting right now!" Ivan now repairs computers and spends his spare time wiring his house to be completely "intelligent" and remote controlled.

Uncovering Your Dream

Christina, the second of fourteen children, was brilliantly talented. Unfortunately, none of her talents could ever be developed because every time she started to do something she was assigned a household chore or another baby was born. Her dream in life was to be a writer, but there was never enough time to write anything more than her homework assignments for her Catholic school, where creativity and spontaneity were not encouraged. Christina grew up to be a jack-of-all-trades, extremely good at beginning projects, or rescuing other people's projects, but unable to focus on her own. She had given up her entire life to help others reach their goals at her expense. In her depression, she began to go for walks. The walks quieted her mind, and she began to remember poems and songs she had written as a child. She realized that, somewhere, her child mind had decided she must not be a good writer because no one ever paid attention to it. Fear of failure surrounded her unavowed dream. She began writing essaylike letters to her friends online. She is now in a writers' group that publishes a literary quarterly.

→ Reconnecting

Whether fear stifled your dream way back in childhood, or it affects your possibilities right now, you first have to discover it. Then you'll be able to see a way to reconnect with your true wishes.

By this time, you probably have an image of yourself from childhood. It may be just in your head, or it may be the image from a photo you still hold on to—that picture of yourself in tutu and tiara, or sitting with a room full of boxes that you turned into a fort. If you have a snapshot, bring it out and place it somewhere visible—on a bulletin board, tacked to the wall, wherever. If there is no photo available, create a picture that evokes your childhood dream. It can be a stick figure. Or a cut-out collage of the elements you associate with it (hammers, wood, and a house, say, if you wanted to be a builder). Each time you look at it, ask yourself, What was/am I afraid of? Sometimes you'll draw a blank, other times something will rise up to your consciousness. Keep your notebook or some sheets of paper nearby and write it down. Over time, you may have collected words like *rejection, abandonment, failure,* even *death.*

As the fears reveal themselves, go back to the appropriate chapters and explore the avenues for getting past those fears. You may also want to read books and look into courses that address your dream, because now you know what has been stopping you!

Part III

Tools and Activities

9. Moving into the World

The suggestions in this chapter range from small beginnings to bold endeavors. Some are quiet, others are physically demanding. Some will invite you to come face-to-face with your fears, others are just plain fun. The one thing they all have in common is that while engaged in any of them, it is extremely difficult to hold on to anxiety about the future.

Each person has different needs and abilities. If you have been suffering from agoraphobia, it's probably not wise to choose martial arts as your first adventure. On the other hand, if you have a tendency to be defensive, or to avoid confrontation, martial arts might be just the thing to help you move forward. Perhaps you have to begin in the privacy of your home with a personal trainer. There is no need to force the issue, to steel yourself with resolve, which will just reinforce the sense of trauma. Review chapter 6 on phobias. If you are afraid to try something you're attracted to, practice the Increasing the Safety Zone exercise starting on page 105 until you're ready to walk into the gym, the movement class, or out on the tennis court.

Fear is one of life's biggest mysteries and challenges. By turning fear into your partner instead of allowing it to be your tormentor, you begin to learn a "dance" that will reveal to you unlimited possibility for self-knowledge and development. In order to fully experience your life, give yourself the gift of self-study. The rewards are immeasurable.

The actions and exercises in part II are personal, often solitary in nature. It is important to spend time with yourself in order to grow. But the opportunities for deeper understanding of your fear can only come from contact with the world you live in. That doesn't mean you have to go in right now and confront your boss and demand a raise, although that time may come. Two things need to happen before then: first, you need to experience your fear while in a safe environment; and, second, you need to experience fear's opposite, the emotions that come from love. Everything you need is right in front of you . . . you just need to recognize it.

Connect with People

Fear often isolates. The ironic thing is that the more you retreat from relationships, the harder it gets to try to have a relationship, any relationship. And the relationships you have become unhealthy. Human beings need relationships in order to survive, not just in the sense that we all depend on each other for goods and services but literally to "relate" to each other. A recent study revealed that children who are not hugged grow up to be learning disabled. They weren't abused; they just weren't loved. If your particular fears have isolated you, you are starving your emotional self. And just like the anorexic who eats less and less, never feeling hungry, you can also lose your appetite for relationships.

Start with one person. Or a group. A church group, for instance, or a book club. Almost anything can begin to bring you back into relationships. Be careful of support groups that are complaint fests where people end up supporting each others' dysfunctions. Find people who are engaged in doing something other than just talking about themselves. Support groups are wonderful for people with diseases who feel alone in their struggle to understand the options available to them and how to work with these options. They are not wonderful when they merely reinforce negative mental attitudes.

Look in your local paper and you'll find everything from groups that discuss films to groups that take walks to groups that pick mushrooms to groups that do volunteer work. The world is eager to meet you.

When you are relating to others—either one on one or in groups—you are experiencing the ultimate benefit of humanity. Animals cannot talk about the meaning of life, let alone the weather. Animals can't dance with each other, let alone practice martial arts. So celebrate your humanity and you will find that love, not fear, joins you along the way.

Learn to Listen

Whether you are alone or with others, learning to listen can lead to a much deeper understanding of your fear and its causes. There are many kinds of listening—some easier and more apparent than others.

Just hearing what other people are saying is a great way to practice listening. It sounds so obvious. Of course I listen, you say. But we don't. You may hear part of the conversation, but at the same time the tapes are rolling in your head. For instance, there's the tape of those things you really want to say in response to what's being said. Sometimes you're so caught up in the tape of your own ideas that you haven't really heard a word the other person is saying. There's that tape playing in the back of your head—the phone call you forgot to make, the little nagging worry about the cyst you found on your arm, your anger at what your mother said to you the other day—all swirling around. And then there's the perhaps unrecognized wish to be someplace else: he talks too much; she's so full of herself; I hate this restaurant. How in the world can you really listen to someone else with all this background noise going on?

Calvin is a successful lawyer with a very busy practice. He was dealing with several clients at the same time, one of them a bothersome old lady who seemed to always show up at his office at the most inopportune moments. He knew her case and her situation, and couldn't be bothered listening to her incoherent ramblings. Then one afternoon, after everyone had left the office, and he was getting ready to go home, she walked in. He was obviously done for the day, no phones were ringing, no more agenda. There was no escape. He sighed and sat down. She began to talk. Calvin decided that instead of staring into space and planning his dinner, he would listen. Suddenly she changed. Instead of a babbling biddy, she was clear, concise, and finished quickly. Shocked, Calvin looked at her. He suddenly realized that all this woman had wanted all along was to be heard. And no one had listened . . . until now.

The benefits of just listening to whomever you're with is that you are truly *there*—not living in your fear story. While you are listening, your head can be clear. It's like exercising a muscle you didn't know you had. You will notice that the person you are speaking to will change, as will your own experience of yourself.

Another way to explore listening is to listen to yourself. It is said that every cell of your body contains all the information of your entire body. Listening is not just with the ears. You know when someone is behind you even without hearing a sound. If you turn your sense of listening inward, you begin to hear/sense profound insights about yourself. Many of the exercises in part II explore this process of inner listening. The more you quiet down, the more you will be able to hear your inner voices of negativity and fear, the more you will sense where your body stores tension and anxiety. Joining a meditation group, or, depending on your faith, a prayer community, can teach you to listen to your inner wisdom.

Use Your Body

One of the best ways to begin to live a courageous life is to engage in activities that require the participation of your body. They are so interesting, so challenging, or just so much fun that there is no space for the voices of fear to gain a foothold. You might say that anytime you are completely involved in something that interests you, you're not thinking about fear anyway. But that's not true. If you are watching TV—be it the news, with stories about anthrax and bombings, or even a soap opera about betrayal and rage—you could be reinforcing your fear beliefs. If you go for a walk with a friend who is always talking about the dangers of parking in the city, you are reinforcing your fear beliefs. If you are gardening but worrying about getting fired, you are reinforcing your fear beliefs.

In some ways, you could say the human body is like the old horse-drawn carriages. They were designed so that as they rumbled along bumpy dirt roads and cobblestone streets, the gears and axles bounced along and lubricated each other. When roads were later paved, the need for lubrication diminished. But then when the carriage would hit a bump a part would break.

Our entire system relies on movement. Vigorous movement increases blood flow, allowing more oxygen to travel through the organism. Endorphins are released, producing a sense of well-being. Varied movements ensure that the joints don't stiffen along a single path, often the cause of injuries and arthritis. Without enough movement, the digestive system becomes sluggish, creating myriad disorders ranging from constipation to cancer. And the less you move, the less you have available to you. As the body becomes brittle and stiff, even walking is approached with trepidation.

Therefore, any kind of movement is going to change your outlook on things. If you have been sitting in your room afraid to move, just taking a walk is a great place to begin. If you are afraid of injuring yourself, find a personal trainer. They are trained to work with every ability level, not just with young jocks with abs of steel.

There is an ancient Eastern saying: "Everything you need to know is contained within your body." I like to think that this means that if I begin to understand what is taking place in my body—the habitual tensions, the unconscious reactions—I can begin to understand more about my psyche. So this effort of getting your body moving is not just throwing yourself into something with all the same habits and attitudes you've carried your whole life; it's a learning process. If you find yourself picking fights on the tennis court, or trying to muscle your partner in judo class, or injuring yourself during tango lessons, listen . . . your body is trying to tell you something about fear. Review some of the lessons in chapter 1 to help identify the core fear behind your negative behavior.

Develop Skills *and* Confidence

> To live with fear and not be afraid is the final test of
> maturity.
> —EDWARD WEEKS

It's true that a person can have wonderful skills and still have tremendous fear. That's one reason why so many talented actors spend their lives waiting tables: the minute they have to present their skills at an audition they freeze up, or they sabotage the audition itself. It's why the best man doesn't always win: the guy with more chutzpah, more networking skills, wins everybody over.

The art of developing confidence could easily take up another book, there are so many approaches and techniques one can practice. From your own body-centered orientation, however, you can begin to develop confidence simply by being more comfortable with yourself. Improving your posture, feeling more ease while moving, knowing how to look someone in the eye while speaking, breathing freely—these "skills" can help you develop the confidence you need to begin reaching outward.

Virginia had taken a course in learning how to "improve her potential" where she was told that each participant had to create a community project. She came up with the innovative idea of getting some local schools to paint a mural on one of the derelict railroad underpasses in the town. She described the idea enthusiastically. All she had to do was call the local high school art teacher and set up a time to "sell" her idea. Weeks went by, and Virginia could not pick up the phone. The time came to report back to her class—now she was doubly terrified. She was going to have to tell a group who had spent weeks "developing her potential" that she couldn't even call the teacher for an appointment. She forced herself over to the phone. As she went to pick it up, she was overwhelmed with nausea and ran vomiting to the bathroom. She had made herself an emotional wreck over a simple call.

Instead of trying to change Virginia's psychology, or trying to analyze her whole life pattern that had led up to this level of insecurity, we tried a simple exercise. All Virginia needed to do was to sense her breath. Each time she felt her breath was constricted, she just needed to pause and wait for it to even out again. As she approached the phone, in fact, Virginia noticed she was holding her breath. She waited. When she picked up the phone, she noticed her breathing becoming rapid and shallow, like a caged animal. She waited again. It took several more days before Virginia actually was able to make the call. But by changing the notion of success from making the call to relaxing the breath, the pressure evaporated. Since then, Virginia has been able to make more calls—both personal and business—without anxiety.

Open Your Heart

Closing yourself off emotionally is one of the negative side effects of fear. When you fear rejection, abandonment, loss, it is easy to drown your feelings—in overwork, television, substance abuse. In previous chapters, we have talked about how emotions can actually impact on your health. When you've been hurt, it often seems logical to shut out troublesome emotions, to just "move on." The problem with this approach is that it doesn't allow joy or love into your heart. When you close yourself off, nothing can penetrate. And without joy in your life, like a flower without light, you will wither away.

There are many avenues to rekindle the life in your heart. Service is one of the safest and best ways to receive what you need. Whether you choose to tutor one child, help in the soup kitchen, or just spend time with someone who is housebound, the reward always outweighs the effort.

Meditation was mentioned earlier as a way to develop listening skills. Engaging in a contemplative discipline also often brings a change of heart. By "sitting" with yourself, or meditating in a group, the mind quiets down, the heart begins to heal.

If sitting still is too daunting, engaging in some movement disciplines can also help. Many people have found that movement, by releasing the body of tension, allows emotions to be more freely expressed. Yoga is the most popular and famous of these disciplines. But there are also many dance groups that use movement to free the emotions.

Gabrielle Roth's Sweat Your Prayers and Dances of Universal Peace, which is an outgrowth of the Sufi community, are just two types available throughout the country. (*See* chapter 10, "Resources.")

Finding the Path

I believe that the existence of the classical "path" can be pregnantly formulated as follows: The "path" comes into existence only when we observe it.

— WERNER HEISENBERG

There's no predicting the outcome of any journey. Werner Heisenberg formulated his famous uncertainty principle based on his frustration trying to predict the path and composition of particles and waves. I remember a cartoon once of a character walking to the moon; as he walked, angels came and placed the flagstones of a path in front of each foot just as he was about to step into the void. In the tarot, the card of the Fool is often illustrated as a man blissfully about to step off a cliff, trusting that the "path" will be there.

It doesn't matter where you begin, because everything is connected and relevant to your journey. You may decide you'd like to start with aikido, because you've always admired martial artists and you figure if you learn to defend yourself you might not be so afraid. Years later, as you deal with a conflict at the office, you find yourself exploring the movement of energy in a relationship instead of hiding in your office afraid to talk to the other party—one of the benefits of aikido. Or you may decide to start doing the Dances of Universal Peace because there's a group in the neighborhood and you haven't danced in years—only to meet a new best friend. The important thing is to begin. Even if you're not sure whether this is really the thing for you.

In a Persian tale, a young man was about to enter a dangerous forest. He was told in no uncertain terms that he had to cross it by nightfall or he would be lost forever. A wise old man who was directing him suggested he use a stick to prod his horse along more quickly on the journey. The young man nodded in agreement, then entered the forest. As the horse meandered, the young man looked for a stick. The first stick he picked up didn't have the right weight. The next stick was too short. A third stick had an awkward grip. So it went through the forest, the young man constantly stopping and examining sticks without being able to choose one. Before he knew it, night had fallen. And he may still be wandering today, because he has never been seen again. It really didn't matter which stick he would have chosen, the important thing was to just choose a stick and get on with it!

10. *Resources*

Some of the activities listed in the preceding chapters may be new to you. Or perhaps you've heard of them but are not sure how they might apply to your needs and interests. This chapter is a resource guide that can help you begin your journey toward a courageous lifestyle in the present. It is not comprehensive, but it gives you a place to begin searching for what works for you. In fact, other activities (chess, book clubs, skydiving, etc.) may better help your development. The emphasis in this guide is on relationship and movement together.

Not everything is available where you live; choose an activity that is local and accessible. On the other hand, there are many things in your own backyard that you may not have even known were there. For those disciplines and explorations that are not as familiar to the general public, definitions are provided, as well as contacts where you can begin your search. Often, a national organization can direct you to a local chapter.

However, there are many classes and offerings available locally that are not part of any national network, and here's where you need to do your own detective work. Local adult and continuing education programs often offer exciting, economical curricula—from ballroom dancing to meditation. Many local hospitals are trying to incorporate mind/body disciplines into their offerings. Your church can be a rich resource of activities. Believe it or not, the Yellow Pages is also loaded with possiblities. And don't hesitate to ask people you know—friends, neighbors, coworkers. The universe can't provide anything unless you ask!

There are some things to look for as you check out places to grow. First of all, is the environment welcoming? Even a high school cafeteria can be welcoming if the people who greet you when you walk in are warm and organized. And yet you can walk into an office that has been feng shuied to within an inch of its life and feel nothing but coldness, condescension, or chaos. Does someone greet you within the first few minutes? Is the atmosphere relaxed? Are the floors clean (especially if the class is on the floor)? Listen to your inner self. Are you turned off because you are nervous and would rather hide? Or is this group genuinely not appropriate for you? When in doubt, give it a second chance. Remember, you are the architect of your experience—not the conditions, but how you respond to these conditions and what you receive from them.

Aikido. Aikido is a martial art called by its founder the "Way of Peace." The literal translation of the name (*ai* = harmony, *ki* = spirit or energy, *do* = way) implies that one works with energy to bring harmony. In aikido, you enter into the attack and blend with the attacker's energy, disarming them, hopefully without hurting them. This discipline involves an in-depth study of skeletal structure and interpersonal dynamics. The result is beautiful and exhilarating. Aikido has no contests; ranks and testing are more for personal growth than ego gratification. There are hundreds of *aikido dojos* (schools) in the world, offering many different styles. The largest group is run by the United States Aikikai Federation: www.usaikifed.com. There are, however, many websites and publications available that can direct you to other schools. (See also Martial Arts, page 159, for other disciplines.)

Ballroom Dancing. Your mother did it, why should you? Because it is a wonderful way to explore relationship without stress. For a few minutes, you are face-to-face with someone. You don't need to speak; just listen to the movement of each other's body. The rhythm of the music combined with learning the discipline of partnered dance steps will increase your coordination and your self-esteem. Try your Yellow Pages, adult schools, or go to www.ballroomdancers.com.

Body-Mind Centering®. Developed by Bonnie Bainbridge Cohen, BMC explores the connection between body and mind using movement, touch, voice, and thought. It is an experiential approach where the student is also the subject:

You study yourself through movement. This method allows you to get deep within all the movements of your body—from the skeletal down to the cellular—in order to develop greater self-knowledge. Go to www.bodymindcentering.com, or contact the School for Body-Mind Centering, 189 Pondview Drive, Amherst, MA 01002-3230; telephone: 413-256-8615.

Chi Kung (or Qigong). This ancient Chinese approach to healing movement has been embraced by the medical community as a safe, complementary discipline for the relief of pain and stress, and for promoting healing. Chi kung exercises can range from very subtle and gentle movements for those with severe pain and limitations to invigorating sequences that are reminiscent of martial arts. Check your local hospital or community center; chances are there is a chi kung group there. Or contact the National Qigong Association for a teacher near you: www.nqa.org.

Dances of Universal Peace. Since the 1960s, the Dances of Universal Peace have touched people around the world. Designed to celebrate the spiritual essence of self, they do not require any dance or movement experience. "Participation, not presentation, is the focus." Go to www.dancesofuniversalpeace.org, or contact the main headquarters at 7400 Sandpoint Way NE, Seattle, WA 98115.

The Feldenkrais Method®. In its mission statement, the Feldenkrais Guild states that the work "transforms people's lives in deep and profound ways, freeing them to enact their avowed and unavowed dreams . . ." Small, relaxing movements explore habits that interfere with optimal functioning and offer new choices for living a fuller life. They can be done by anyone and require no movement experience. See the appendix, page 165, for more information. Or go to www.feldenkrais.com; telephone: 800-775-2118.

Folk Dancing. For millennia, people have gathered together to dance the spirit of their heritage, from Irish step dancing to flamenco. The steps of each country echo with history. As you hop to a Polish Krakoviak, or stamp in an Indian Kathak dance, you are participating in a ritual that has enriched countless lives and literally held societies together. This feeling is still there, each time a group gathers to exchange the steps of its people. And even though many of the dances are not partner dances, all of them involve relationship and connection in order to work. Go to www.folkdancing.org, or contact the Folk Dance Association, P.O. Box 30500, Brooklyn, NY 11230; telephone: 718-434-1766.

Martial Arts. There are dozens of ways to explore the art of self-defense—from the meditative quality of tai chi, through aikido (see listing on page 157) to more confrontational arts like kung fu and tae kwon do. When looking for a martial arts school, you need to decide what works for you. Some things to verify before you sign up at a school:

1. Who are the teachers? What is their experience, training, rank (if there is rank)?
2. What is the behavior on the mat/floor? Do partners treat each other with respect or with aggression?
3. What is the emphasis at the school—competition and results, or compassion and learning? Some clues: if the school is crowded with trophies and contest announcement/enrollment forms, you're dealing with a competitive, commercial enterprise. Notice how large their retail section is. What is the décor? Pictures of their sensei with celebrities and trophies? Or flower arrangements and simple designs?
4. What is the cleanliness factor?

Here are just a few sites: for kung fu, www.kungfuonline. com or www.shaolin.com; for U.S. tae kwon do, www.ustu. com; for tai chi, www.taichi.com.

Meditation. Although meditation is considered a solitary experience, it can still be extremely helpful in working with fear, especially in a group setting. There are many forms of meditation available, each with a slightly different style. You may find that only one or two are available in your area, or that there is a bewildering array of styles to choose from. Begin with any one of them—it certainly can't hurt you. As Lao-tse said, "A journey of a thousand miles begins with a single step." Some approaches to investigate: Insight Meditation (Vipassana), www.dharma.org; 1230 Pleasant Street,

Barre, MA 01005, telephone: 978-355-4378; Zen, www. zencenter.org; Transcendental Meditation, www.tm.org, telephone: 888-LearnTM.

NIA. Described as a synthesis of dance, martial arts, and Feldenkrais (see appendix, page 165), NIA stands for *Neuromuscular Integrative Action*. NIA dance stresses the connection among body, mind, and spirit. Each class offers students an opportunity to explore themes like centering, gravity, flow, stability, etc. Students learn very simple routines done to an eclectic program of music designed to inspire. Teachers are carefully trained, earning belts like in the martial arts as they grow in experience. Go to www.nia-nia.com.

Waves. Described by some as ecstatic dance, founder Gabrielle Roth calls it "sweating your prayers." Using tribal/trance music, participants express themselves in free dance that explores qualities like fluidity and chaos. It is a shared group discipline that requires no experience. Go to www.gabrielleroth.com.

Conclusion: Love Is Being in the Present

ear is part of the human experience. Even Jesus Christ, on the night of his arrest, begged God to relieve him of what was to come. We live in a universe where we need hot to know cold, pain to know pleasure, war to feel peace. However, no one needs to live in fear. No one needs to be a victim of fear. Instead, fear can become your teacher. The minute you are experiencing fear, you can be sure that you are no longer living in the present moment. As was said earlier, fear only appears when you are expecting something to happen, living in the future, often based on your past experience.

On the other end, love can only be experienced in the present moment. Thinking about past love, imagining a future love, isn't love. That incredible sense of spontaneity, the joyful quality of play—whether it's with someone or in the midst of a task—this is the experience of love.

You cannot "will" yourself to feel love. But you can make efforts to be more present. When you feel fear, anxiety, or the emotions that mask fear—be it anger, sadness, or even boredom—you have a built in reminder that you are not present. All of the exercises in this book are ways to help you recognize this fact.

Learning to live in the present moment is a life's work, perhaps it is even "the work" that we need to do before we become self-realized individuals. So don't get discouraged as you explore your habits, your fears, your world. You have nothing to lose but fear itself.

Appendix: What Is the Feldenkrais Method®?

Born in Russia in 1904, Dr. Moshe Feldenkrais lived most of his life in Israel. An engineer, scientist, and athlete, Feldenkrais was determined to recover from debilitating knee pain that began with a soccer injury. In studying infant development, brain function, animal movement, and more, he discovered several principles that helped him walk again. His first book, *Body and Mature Behavior,* appeared in 1947, and his last, *The Potent Self,* in 1985, the year after his death. Over this course of time, Dr. Feldenkrais applied his method to athletes, musicians, people with severe disabilities, children with birth defects, and even politicians (he taught David Ben-Gurion to stand on his head!). His study for the potential in human learning brought him into contact with some of the greatest minds of our time: Yehudi Menuhin,

Margaret Mead, Gregory Bateson, were just a few of his admirers.

Many of Moshe Feldenkrais's ideas have become part of the new field of somatic education. They include:

- The human organism is a system. What affects one part affects the whole.
- The nervous system learns through movement, repetition, and rest in a safe environment.
- Our behavior is the result of habits developed over a lifetime. Developing awareness of these habits can improve quality of life.
- At each moment, four things are happening: thinking, feeling, sensing, and movement. Yet most people live in only one part at a time. The Feldenkrais Method helps develop awareness of the other parts.

The Feldenkrais Method is taught according to three general principles:

- Less is more. It is not the size of your movement but the quality of your attention that leads to improvement.
- Stay within your comfort level. Feldenkrais said, "Learning should be a pleasurable experience. If you are not enjoying yourself, you are not learning."
- Rest whenever necessary.

Further Reading

Julia Cameron, *The Artist's Way* (New York: Tarcher/Putnam, 1992).

Joseph Campbell, *The Masks of God* (New York: Arkana, 1995).

Deepak Chopra, M.D., *Quantum Healing* (New York: Bantam Books, 1990).

Norman Cousins, *Anatomy of an Illness* (New York: Bantam Books, 1991).

Dalai Lama, *An Open Heart* (Boston: Little, Brown, 2002).

Antonio Damasio, *The Feeling of What Happens* (San Diego: Harcourt, 2000).

———, *Descartes' Error* (New York: Avon Books, 1995).

Moshe Feldenkrais, *The Potent Self* (Berkeley, Calif.: Frog Ltd., 2002).

———, *Awareness Through Movement* (San Francisco: Harper, 1991).

Jack Kornfield, *A Path with Heart* (New York: Bantam, 1993).

Gary Kraftsow, *Yoga for Wellness* (New York: Arkana, 1999).

Lao-tzu, Jonathan Star, *Tao Te Ching: The Definitive Edition* (New York: Tarcher/Putnam, 2001).

Caroline Myss, Ph.D., *Anatomy of the Spirit* (New York: Harmony Books, 1996).

Joseph Chilton Pearce, *The Biology of Transcendence* (Rochester, Vt.: Park Street Press, 2002).

Candace Pert, Ph.D., *Molecules of Emotion* (New York: Simon & Schuster, 1999).

Don Miguel Ruiz, *The Four Agreements* (San Rafael, Calif.: Amber-Allen, 1997).

Idris Shah, *World Tales* (London: Octagon Press, 1991).

Michael Talbot, *The Holographic Universe* (New York: Harper-Perennial, 1992).

Eckhart Tolle, *The Power of Now* (Novato, Calif.: New World Library, 1999).

Index

About the Author

An Emmy-nominated choreographer and former artist-in-residence at the Guggenheim Museum in New York City, Lavinia Plonka is a longtime teacher and student of movement practices with experience on the stage, in classrooms, and on television. A master teacher/performer of mime and mask, she continues to consult, choreograph, and perform around the world. Blending her disciplines, Plonka teaches workshops throughout the country that explore issues such as fear, creativity, mythology, and body language. She lives in North Carolina, where she maintains a successful Feldenkrais practice. You can visit her website at www.laviniaplonka.com.